CONFINEMENT CHRONICLES

Encouraging Testimonies Birthed Out of the 2020 Pandemic

Stories Compiled by Angie BEE Productions

Edited by Zaundra George

for

ƠNSPIRED™

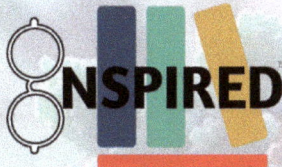

Reading for the Whole Person

INSPIRED published by
Ladero Press LLC
229 Kettering Road
Deltona, Florida 32725

First Ladero Press Printing, July 2021

Confinement Chronicles:
Encouraging Testimonies Birthed Out of the 2020 Pandemic

ISBN: 978-1-946981-70-7 Paperback / 978-1-946981-71-4 EPUB /
978-1-946981-72-1 Mobi

Printed in the United States of America
Set in Times New Roman
Cover Designed by SheerGenius

TABLE OF CONTENTS

ACKNOWLEDGEMENTS

This project has been the result of sponsors and individuals lending their gifts and talents. We could not have seen the audiobook come to fruition without them.

Thank you to the authors for taking time to put your thoughts on paper during such a challenging time. You answered the call, and I'm thankful.

Thank you to Theresa Jordan of *Triumphant Magazine* for promoting this project in your magazine. Your support has surely helped our message reach the masses.

Thank you to Donna M. Gray-Banks of F.R.E.S.H. Book Festival for your promotional support and e-mail blasts.

Thank you to my family for your love and support, during the completion of this project.

Finally, a sincere shout out of appreciation to DJ Shyheim of HalfTime Productions and Rapture Beats for providing several of the background tracks used in this project. We are grateful for your gifts and talents.

INTRODUCTION

When the Lord first instructed me to produce an inspirational audiobook, I never dreamed that authors from far-and-wide would contribute to this project! As they continued to send us their stories, I slowly began to realize that all of these stories would not fit in a sixty-minute audio! Why the sixty-minute specification? Well, although we are now in the age of MP3 players, there are still people who want to listen to a compact disc, and CDs can hold up to sixty minutes of audio. I was thinking small; God showed me HIS bigger picture.

After the call for submissions went out, stories began to pour in. Soon after, we had enough stories to fill not only Volume I, but Volume II, and even Volume III. The posted deadline for submissions was June 1st, and it was only May 20th! I was still waiting on contributions from three more people! LOOK AT GOD!

Now, I understand that the *Confinement Chronicles* will never end; just like the Word of God never grows old. Each volume evolved into something more that God desired to communicate. There are *Confinement Chronicles* of our minds and our relationships. There are *Confinement Chronicles* of our finances and our "lack of faith." In one-way-or-another, these inspirational audiobooks will continue to encourage us to hear the Word of God; they will encourage us to write; and they will encourage us to share.

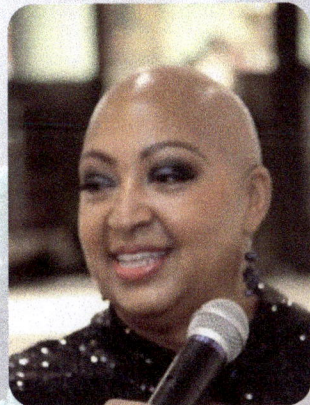

As we introduce the complete written adaptation of the popular audiobook series, we encourage you to order the audiobooks to complement this printed version. We encourage you to prepare yourself for a delight that your mind will not soon forget!

Enjoy and BEE Blessed!

Sincerely,

Evangelist Angie BEE

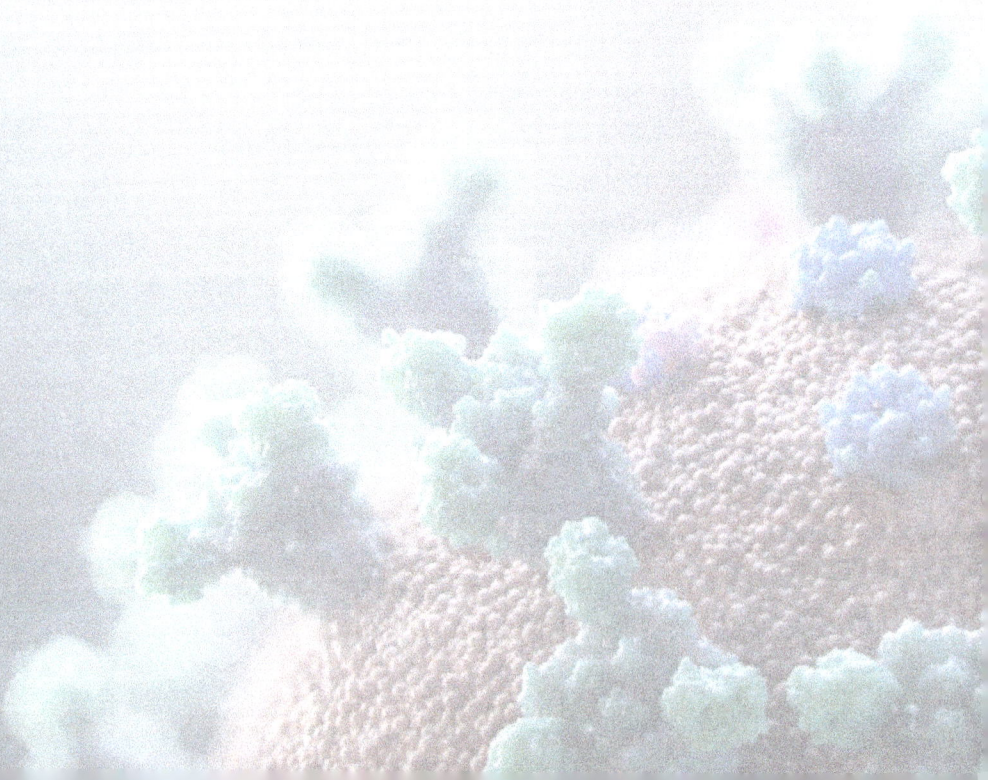

CONFINEMENT CHRONICLES

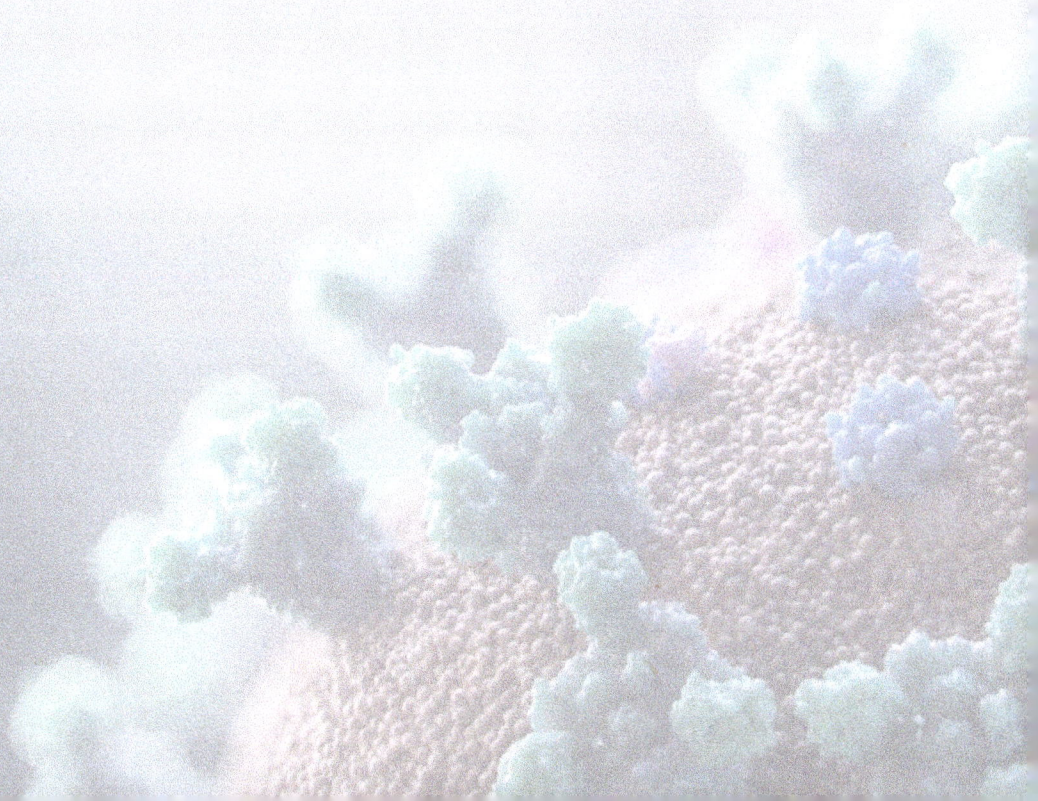

VOLUME I

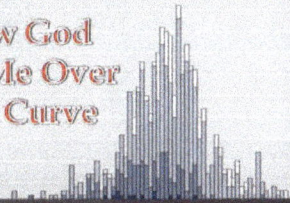

Confinement Chronicles

How God Got Me Over The Curve

Encouraging Testimonies Birthed from the 2020 Coronavirus Pandemic

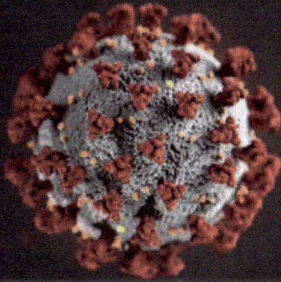

An inspirational audiobook compilation series
Produced by

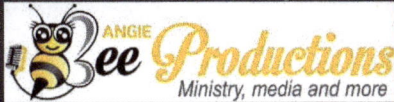

ANGIE Bee Productions
Ministry, media and more

BEFORE, DURING OR AFTER?

Getting Through COVID-19

Neka Perkins

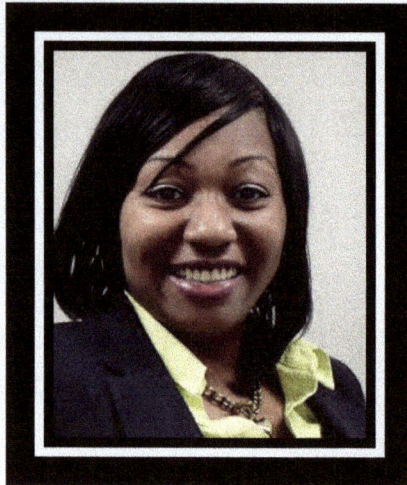

It was one night in March and I headed to bed as I normally would.
A shower, a prayer to the Man, and ready to enjoy a good night's sleep as everyone should.

Woke up the next morning and the T.V. was tuned in on the news.
Hearing all the chatter about the spread of COVID-19 and suddenly I became confused.

I continued to lie in bed while saying to myself, "This must be a dream."
Realizing more as they chattered, it was exactly what it seemed.

Fox 5 San Diego News and the rest of the world were suddenly up in arms
Delivering the spreading news of COVID-19 was making everyone alarmed.
Soon we would learn the stores and schools would shutdown
The crowds would soon disappear making the busy streets appear like a ghost town.

No more trips to the grocery store without wearing gloves and mask
Not knowing how I would adjust to the new normal was in itself a challenging task.

With a first grader at home, quickly transitioning the family room into a classroom
The new technological advances were a blur and just like that I was utilizing Zoom.

Taking random breaks to regroup and reorganize throughout the busy day
Often explaining to an active six-year-old, "why things were now this way."

All while keeping my trust and faith where it always belonged
Striving to keep a positive perspective and praying for His protection all the day long.

Tuning into Sunday online church services and especially for Easter
Realizing this moment in time was indeed a chance for a quick breather.

A quick breather to keep important things into perspective with my family as the main focus
I was no longer trying to understand why we were suddenly "stuck" in this new locus.

Realizing more and often that everything has a purpose because God always has a plan
So much so, He controls everything including COVID-19 because the whole world is in his hands.
In this moment of trial and test, one has to decide will they grow closer or farther away
I choose to grow nearer because COVID won't always be here to stay.

When God moves his hand and calls all his people home
We will all then realize He never left us alone.

Some people feel very lonely, some people are super afraid
But we must get rid of all of those unknown anxieties and give our Father more sincere praise.

Even in these trying times, He simply wants us to trust Him more
So much so, I was even forced to look inside---deeply at my core.

Although life after COVID-19 won't exactly be the same
God is the same God and He's always handing out His mercy and grace.

Truth be told, we can still live life full of hope, faith, positivity and laughter.
So, as we continue to fight the good fight, will you focus on the before, the during or the after?

Quarantine Chronicles

Three, Short Compilations from A Single Mother That Is Quarantined with Her Only Child During This Pandemic of 2020

Sonya Bennett

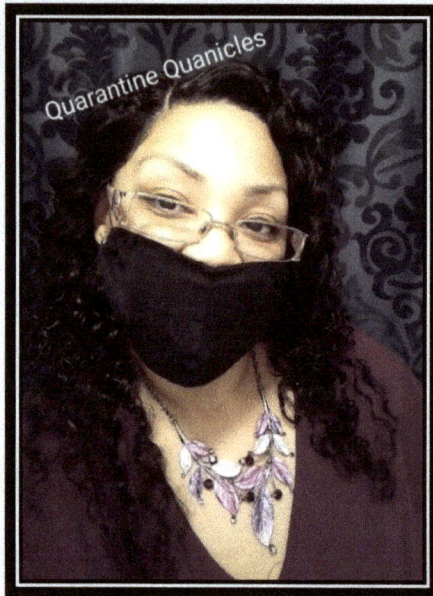

Story I - Google Who?

It's Day 313 of the pandemic quarantine in Detroit, Michigan. It's something how this started as a minor inconvenience: schools are closed today <u>and</u> tomorrow? Guess it will be a four-day weekend.

Little did I know...

We started hearing terms we aren't used to: N-95 Masks, pandemic, quarantine, social-distancing, Google School -- wait, what? No more 'building' school? Parents are not only working from home, but now we are assisting teachers in the learning process from home?   Once passively-completed homework is now mandatory-schoolwork <u>from</u> home? Okay: well, let's get to our new "normal."

English, Math, Social Studies for a second grader; how hard could it be? Sure, I'm a spry forty-nine that -- in these eight years – I've taught her to walk, talk, potty-train and independently think, so this should be a piece of cake!

You're sleepy? What? You stayed awake in school, didn'tcha?

Wait: didn't her teacher send home notes about her falling asleep in class? I politely replied, "I'll put her to bed earlier."

Hey: stay focused! You've only done an hour of work: why are you on a video chat?

Wait: didn't her teacher mention in parent-teacher conferences that she sloppily rushes through her work so that she may draw, giggle, and socialize with other distracted peers?

Damn: lemme send a fruit basket to her teacher. *Wait: the school 'building' is closed - duh!* It will have to be a virtual gift card for Educator Appreciation Week because this struggle is REAL!

In 2021, I will have an entirely new appreciation for Educators: sanitizers, school supplies, bathroom tissue, ... and you need me to volunteer my time? No problem!! I will come in for a full day, and I will be rolling a monogrammed suitcase with your initials on it, filled with all of those items that you like— hoping that you take that suitcase on a much-deserved vacation!

Miss y'all

THE GAME CHANGER

Monique A. Chandler

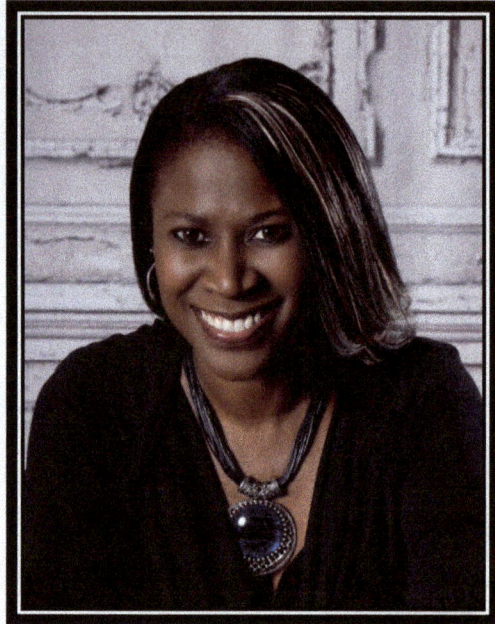

The year was 2002; spring was the season, and March Madness was in full swing. My older sister, Lisa—my beautiful, brilliant, and loving shero— was bravely fighting a losing battle with liver disease, and my heart was breaking. From the time I was a little girl, I looked up to my sister. Not only was she very pretty, but she was kind. She had such a gentle spirit that I don't think she made one enemy in her lifetime. Lisa was the type of person who painstakingly built all of her relationships with love and honesty. Not only did I love her, I actually liked her as a person and loved being able to tell people she was MY big sister.

Even though we were four years apart, Lisa and I shared a love for sports. We would spend all of our free time discussing basketball and football. If we weren't talking about sports, we were watching them on television or in-person. Lisa and her best friend, Veronica Johnson, would often let me tag along with them to basketball or football games. Roni, as Veronica was affectionately known, was much like Lisa; she had a lot of associates who wanted to become friends. Veronica and Lisa somehow developed a comfortable sisterhood that was so honest and true, that Lisa made Veronica promise if anything ever happened to her, that Veronica would take care of me; become a surrogate big sister.

Every year in March, Lisa and I would get into these intense discussions on which college teams would make it to the "Sweet Dance" and the NCAA Men's Final Four. During the tournaments we would challenge each other on which teams would advance in the college brackets. For years, we looked forward to our March Madness traditions because we had so much fun teasing and debating with each other . . . Until it all came to an abrupt halt in the spring of 2002.

As greatly as we wanted to, we couldn't do much debating because Lisa was not feeling well. I remember going to see her in Jacksonville and arriving to her house late at night. As I dozed in the chair beside Lisa's bed, I was awakened by her soft voice.

"Mo, I have three wishes for my life," she whispered.

I sat up in the chair and shook my head quickly to ward off sleep. "Three wishes," I repeated groggily. "What are they?" I asked quietly.

Lisa smiled warmly as her eyes welled up with tears. "I trust that God allows me to see my fortieth birthday," she said while holding up one finger. Her birthday was three and a half weeks away. "I trust that my son will get a scholarship to college." She raised two fingers. Her son had been waiting to hear back from the college of his choice regarding his scholarship application. "And finally, I trust that you, my little sister, will be the one to find my first strand of gray hair." Lisa laughed as she held up three fingers and stared at me with a resigned look in her eyes.

My heart felt like it would break into a thousand pieces because it was at that moment, I realized my sister was facing her own mortality, but I wasn't ready to face the possibility. I hugged Lisa tightly and told her, "God's got you, Sis, and we've got each other."

A few weeks later I received a call from Mom. I remember it was the first week in April, and I was at work. "Lisa is in the hospital in Gainesville," Mom said solemnly.

Immediately, I informed Gigi, my supervisor, and I got into my car and left work. I didn't go home to pack a bag or call anyone to let them know what was going on. I just got into my car and began the long drive from Buford, Georgia, to Gainesville, Florida. In hindsight, I don't know how I made it because I was driving on autopilot. I was alone in my car; alone with my thoughts, and that was not a good place to be. My mind was stayed on Lisa. How was I going to go on without my big sister? Who was going to encourage me to fulfill my dreams, and who was going to debate me about college basketball? I didn't want my nephew to have to grow up without his mother, and I was worried about the impact Lisa's illness was having on my mom.

I arrived in Gainesville around two AM and planned to see Lisa first thing in the morning, but that was not to be. The doctor called Mom and told her they were transporting Lisa by air to Hospice of Jacksonville. I was confused. I didn't know why they were transporting her, but I made myself believe they wanted her to be near family so she could reap the benefits of the family's tender loving care.

I honestly did not know what Hospice Care was about, but I could look at my mom and see that she was numb. Her eyes held a sadness that I had never seen before, and I felt completely helpless. I needed someone to explain Hospice Care to me, and I needed Mom to smile and tell me that everything was going to be okay -- that Lisa was going to be okay. But again, that was not to be.

I watched my mom stare out the car window as we made the 45-minute ride to Jacksonville. I wanted to say something that would take her pain away, but I couldn't find the words. All I could do was stand by helpless as my sister lay unconscious, and my mother sat heartbroken.

"Aunt Di," I cried into the phone. "I'm here at the hospital with Mom. Lisa is sick, and I don't know what to do. Mom isn't talking, and I don't know what to say to make her feel better." Tears were rolling down my face as I listened to Aunt Di's soothing voice. I don't remember what she said to me on that day, all I know was her tone was comforting, and I drew strength from across the miles.

We had been at Hospice a few minutes, and a doctor came out to speak with us. I was listening to him explain what was to be their role in Lisa's transition, and I sat quietly listening to every heartbreaking word, determined to be strong for Lisa and my mom.

"May I see my sister?" I asked the doctor afterward.

"Yes, you can," he replied. "We've given her some morphine to help ease her discomfort as she transitions," he said, "but you may sit with her."

I walked into the room, and the only thing I could think about was Lisa's three wishes. I kept hearing her voice over and over again telling me she trusted that she would make it to her fortieth birthday on April 7th; her son would get a college scholarship; and I would find her first strand of gray hair. My head began to spin, and my breathing accelerated. I ran out of the room and made it to the restroom right before my body was wracked by a severe panic attack.

A few hours later, two doctors came to speak with us to explain the dying process to our family. Lisa was settled in resting peacefully. I went into her room and noticed that someone had brushed her long hair back neatly and put it into a ponytail. As I walked around her bed, I rubbed Lisa's beautiful face. As I brushed back a few stray hairs, I noticed one long, shiny gray hair.

"Mom, look," I whispered excitedly. I motioned for all of my relatives to come and look at Lisa's gray strand. When I got a few peculiar stares, I realized that I was the only one who knew about Lisa's three wishes.

As we sat around her room, my nephew walked in. He walked up to his mother's bed and kissed her gently on the forehead. My heart broke for him because I knew it would be hard going on without his mother. He looked over at me and Mom and smiled sadly before taking a deep breath.

"I will be headed to college in the fall," he said proudly. "I'm going to FAMU on a scholarship!" He'd received the news.

My breath caught in my throat, and tears came to my eyes as I realized that two of Lisa's wishes had been fulfilled. I looked over at my sister and said a silent prayer for her. Tomorrow was to be her birthday, but tomorrow was not promised to her.

I chose to believe Lisa would live to see her birthday, and so I planned a surprise birthday celebration for her. I called Publix and ordered a cake and invited our relatives to come and celebrate with us. Lisa's born day emerged beautifully; everything was gloriously green and butterflies fluttered outside of her window. I remember looking out at the brilliant sunlight and thanking God for sparing my sister's life and fulfilling her last wishes. We picked up the cake, and for a moment, I just stared down at the words on it that read: *"Happy Birthday, Lisa. We Love You!"*

Happy Birthday to you. Happy Birthday to you. Happy Birthday, Dear Lisa. Happy Birthday to Youuuu. How old are you? How old are you? How old are you? How old are you? She's 40 years old. She's 40 years old. She's 40 years old. SHE'S 40 YEARS OLD!!!

We softly sang the birthday song to Lisa, and I remember thinking I had never heard anything so beautiful. Lisa, my beautiful, brilliant, loving big sister had lived to see her fortieth birthday; thus, fulfilling her three wishes. I remember looking down at Lisa's pretty face and thinking that she must have been pleased, because she had the most peaceful smile on her face. Although I was grief stricken, I was happy and proud once again to tell the world that she was MY big sister.

I had to leave later on that night because I had a mandatory inspection at work the next morning. I didn't hit the road until after eight PM, and I knew I had a long trip back to Atlanta. As soon as I got into the car, I began to cry. I cried and I cried until I was all cried out. By that time, my eyes were severely swollen. I could barely see out of them and decided to exit the interstate and grab a cup of coffee. I sat in my car in the Waffle House parking lot for a few minutes, trying to get myself together before I walked in and ordered a coffee.

My waitress looked at me with concern, asking if I was all right. I told her I was and then walked to the restroom to check my appearance. I looked ghastly. My eyes looked like I had been on the losing end of a heavyweight boxing match. I vaguely remember seeing a bunch of bikers as I exited the restroom. I grabbed my coffee and walked to my car. Once I made it to my car, I sat behind the wheel and a dam broke inside of me. My heart began aching as I poured out all of my grief. I banged on the steering wheel as I cried out Lisa's name and prayed. I rested my head on the steering wheel as my tears began to dissipate, but then reality set in that I could barely see, and I had to get back to Atlanta by morning.

I heard a rapping on the driver's side window. I looked up to see the waitress.

"Are you okay, Sweetie?" she asked through the window. I looked behind her and saw a bunch of bikers clad in leather vests and jeans. I was too distraught to worry about whether or not I was in harm's way. I rolled down the window a little bit and the waitress asked again if I was okay.

"My sister is in hospice in Jacksonville, and I have to get back to Atlanta for an inspection at work," I cried while shaking my head hopelessly.

One of the bikers came to my window and replied, "Listen, young lady. I have a daughter, and I would want someone to help her if she was having difficulty getting home." The other bikers nodded their assent in the background. "Where do you live in Atlanta?" he asked.

I answered that I lived off the Mall of Georgia exit. One of the other bikers acknowledged that he knew where that exit was, and then, shortly thereafter, we were on our way.

For over three hours I was surrounded by a dozen bikers on Harley Davidson motorcycles. They surrounded my car as I drove back to Atlanta, until I put my right turn signal on at Exit 115 off 85 North in Buford, Georgia. Once I exited, they did a U-turn and blew their horns at me. I drove into Preston Hills at Mill Creek Apartments at seven AM. on Monday morning. I ran inside to quickly prepare for work and had just sat on the side of my bed when the cell phone on my nightstand rang. My heartbeat accelerated because deep in my heart I already knew . . .

"She just left us," Mom's sad voice said on the other end.

My sister, Lisa, transitioned on April 8, 2002, and we celebrated her Home Going Service on April 13 with heavy hearts.

Every year since then, I honor Lisa's love for college basketball by watching March Madness and attending the NCAA Women's Final Four. It was our mutual love for college basketball that bonded us and gave me a way to celebrate Lisa in a manner that I know is pleasing to her. Before her passing, I loved the moments Lisa and I spent together, but her death became a game changer for me. Now, March Madness is not just about the game of basketball. It's a reminder of the special bond I shared with my brilliant, beautiful and kind big sister, Lisa. And it's a reminder to always celebrate life today, for it's not promised to us tomorrow.

TROUBLE DON'T LAST ALWAYS

Theresa Jordan

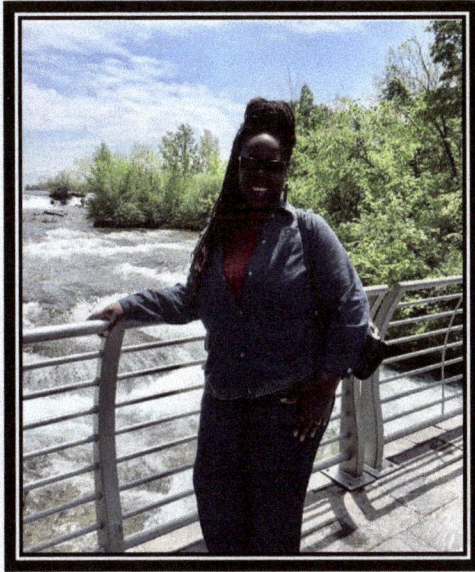

W e do not have to wait for this pandemic to be finished to give our Lord all the honor and glory due to Him. He deserves our praises, so don't wait for the battle to be over. Because we have already won, and the victory belongs to Jesus. We serve a God that is wiser, stronger, and bigger than our circumstances. I love the song that Hezekiah Walker sings, "Every Praise." It is a constant reminder that no matter what we are going through, God still deserves the praise.

The Lord promised in Isaiah 26:3 - *Thou wilt keep him in perfect peace, whose mind is stayed on thee because he trusteth in thee.* I am grateful that the Lord blesses us with peace, and it's the peace that only He can give. (Numbers 6:24-26) says, *The LORD bless thee, and keep thee: The LORD make his face shine upon thee, and be gracious unto thee: The LORD lift up his countenance upon thee, and give thee peace.*

The amazing part is the blessings we are receiving did not start with you and me, but God's blessings and mercy extend from generation to generation. Our mothers, grandmothers, and great-grandmothers knew Him as a Way maker. The children of Israel knew the Lord as a way maker; therefore, it is our responsibility to let others know He will do the same for them. He is more than capable of making a way out of no way at all.

We serve a God that is a keeper. I love Psalm 121 (the entire chapter) verse 5: *The Lord is they keeper: the Lord is thy shade upon thy right hand.* I heard this philosophy years ago, and over the years, it has become my philosophy, "God said it, I believe it, and that settles it."

He is a promise keeper. How do I know? Because He is not a man that He should lie, and I know there is nothing too hard for God. I have personally witnessed it first-hand for myself over the years, and I know that what is impossible through man is possible through God.

Once this pandemic is over and it will be.......

Please remember (Psalm 103:2) – *Bless the Lord, O my soul, and forget not all his benefits.* A Pastor preached a sermon one day, and she reminded the church that we shouldn't forget the Lord's benefits and the things He has done and things He continues to do in our lives. My desire is to always be like the one leper that remembered to come back and give the Lord all the glory, praises, and honor due to Him. When, on the other hand, the other 9 lepers did not return, and some might say, it was because they were ungrateful. I want to remember and to always be grateful for all of my blessings.

Remember trouble don't last always, and this too shall pass!

7 WAYS GOD GOT ME OVER THE CURVE DURING A WORLD CRISIS

Excerpts from the Upcoming Book

Rue Mayweather

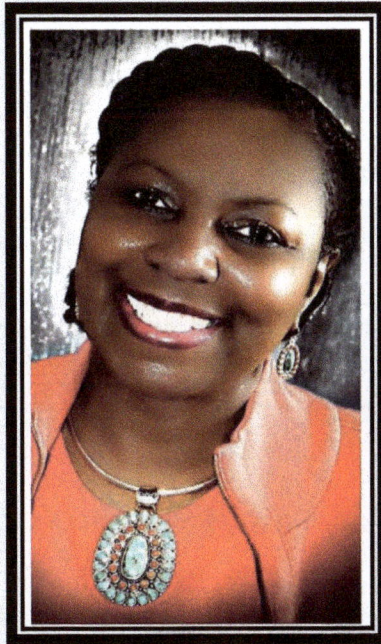

1. Four Critical Elements
Sleep Hygiene, Nutrition, Physically Active and Social Support

These four critical elements go hand-in-hand when the body is combating a virus of any kind. One part affects the other. Not getting enough sleep will cause you to feel lackadaisical which affects your energy level, and you may skimp on having a well-balanced meal and eat something not as nutritious. This, in turn, makes you feel sluggish and not active and definitely feel anti-social. Having a strong social support system during a time of pandemic or crisis is golden, especially if family or friends aren't able to visit you in person.

2. Take Breaks from the News

Although I am a news junkie, I took a break from the news--from a ritual of three, sometimes, four times a day, and treated myself to a date every night with none other than the judicial prince himself, Perry Mason. The joke between us, unbeknownst to him, was to determine who could determine the outcome of the case first. I usually won. Using this method as a break from news was great. It gave me something to look forward to, although I had to stay up later in the evening for my date. Wait, Wait, Wait! Perry Mason didn't tell me; however, I found out that I could also have coffee with him every day Monday through Friday at eight o'clock in the morning.

3. Make Time to Unwind

Making time to unwind isn't as difficult for me as it may be for most. During my thirty-plus years in the military, I didn't realize how busy and how fast my speedometer was going until I stopped. Then, I had an "Oh My" moment. I love music, therefore, at any given time, you may hear me listening to some really nice jazz or singing some really great gospel music. Praying and speaking in tongues never gets old for me. Sometimes, I don't know what to say or pray about. I simply get on my knees or lie flat and let all of the world's issues flow to Him.

Don't become afraid of what you don't know. The population for which facts seem to be air in the wind is our young generation – maybe because they don't watch the news, or they seek their facts from a different source (invalidated): a source that allows them to believe that they are all right, and this virus cannot and will not compromise their system because they are young and virile. Fact, we must let them know that there are other people in the world who can be affected and guess what? They, these young and virile people, can be the carriers, who transmit this virus to an older loved one without knowing they – in-fact—are the carrier and kill them. Fact.

4. Not Waiting to See if Older People Need Assistance

Something in the air or wind with this virus has brought out the goodness and kindness in all of us. Not sure if we think if God sees if we tried to do just a little bit of good while he watched us during this last quarter it would account for something, but we tried. I really needed water and couldn't find any. I finally was able to purchase four large bottles at the dollar store. Although, I wasn't trying to do a lot of moving around and being in large crowds. Having my eighty-six-year-old aunt out and about to shop was definitely out. Knowing that she could use some essential items such as tissue, Pine Sol, and paper towels, I was able to find a store that had a fresh supply with no limit and purchased it for her so she wouldn't have to worry about running out. Another act of kindness for seniors is that if you see any in line to please allow them the courtesy of going first. I don't know about you, but I am not really used to waiting in very long lines. With the pandemic, good Lord, sometimes the lines seem to stretch from here to never as the saying goes. This is the same with the self-check-out counters, as well.

5. Feeling Peace in Chaos

Whereas I knew there was a lot of chaos surrounding the virus, I also felt peace about it. I was deeply aware that the virus was a silent killer, and I, like most, was not exempt. I had come close to death so many times. I am grateful for each new day. True, I have no idea what will take me out and, like most who received their angel wings via the coronavirus and had no idea they would, I don't know either.

6. Praying No Longer About Me

I believe there is power in prayer. Prayer is an action word followed by faith. I find myself praying more for others than myself. I recall not having a job and having to look for one. To see the long line of people needing food is no joke. Some people are picky about what they eat. Most of us will experience a juncture in our lives when we become grateful to have food. I will certainly do it for others when I see they need help without them having to ask. With so many of the things we're used to not being available to us, prayer is the least that we have yet the greatest gift that we can offer everyone sincerely with no limit. It's as if the world has been turned upside down, and there's no way to upend it again. Yes, I need prayer more than ever, especially since the virus seems to just hang a limb or in mid-air waiting to drop at will on the next unsuspecting person. Yet, I pray for others, as well. I am blessed to be able to go in and shelter in place or wash my hands for twenty seconds, or if need be, take my temperature. There are those who are not. Life from this perspective seems like a small fare. We know it isn't. Those who are incarcerated and trafficked consume my prayers most. I know for most they do not have the luxury of privacy to escape from the virus. The idea of a bleach-sanitized environment may be out of the question for them.

7. Investing in Self

Even in this pandemic, I will use my old cliche of "don't give all of yourself away." Manage your body like you manage your tithe – the first part goes to God, then the other portion to yourself. What's remaining goes to others. Take care of yourself so you'll have something left to give to others: be it time, money, or something else. It's really difficult to let ourselves go especially now that we're stuck inside. Get up; open the windows; let the sunshine in; sing a song; put some makeup on.

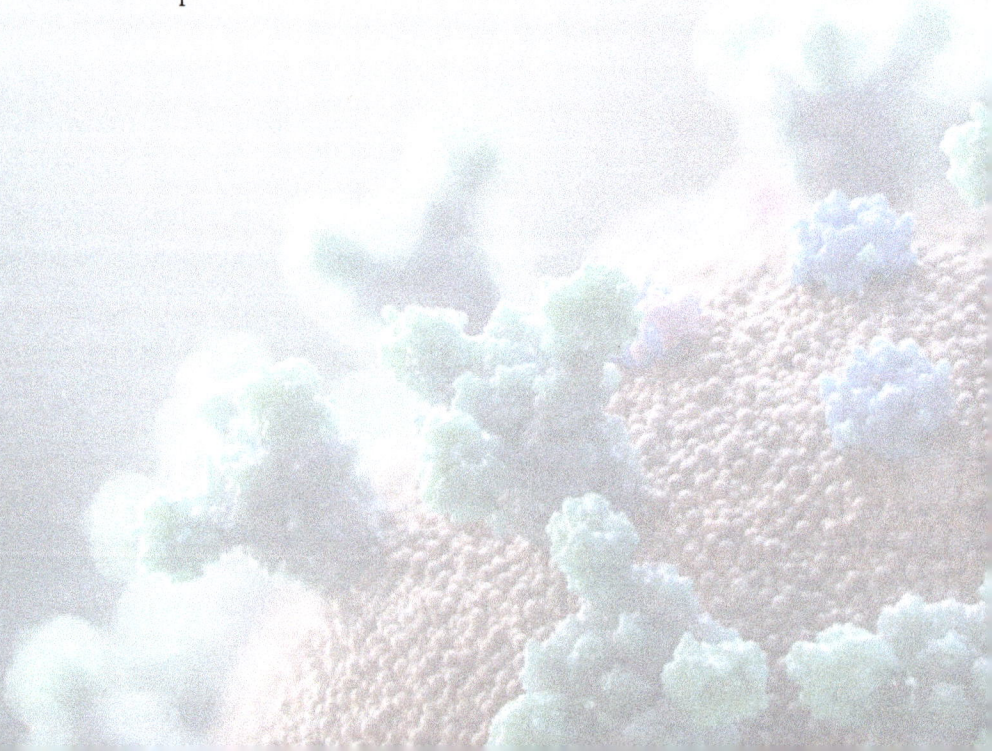

THE BEST PARTY EVER!

Terri Jones

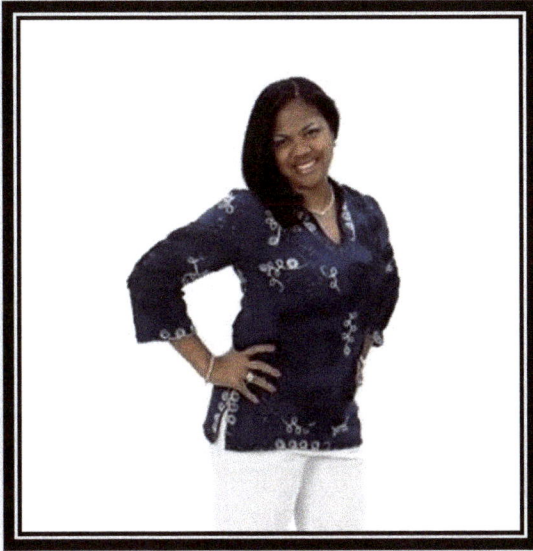

As a woman of God, author, teacher and techie during the coronavirus pandemic, I chose to continue to do what I was put on this earth to do: tap into my God-given creativity.

It was a month before Chrisette's birthday when her mom received an email notification from the local school she was attending. The parents and students were informed of the decision to close the school because of the coronavirus call to practice social distancing. *Oh, no*, I thought. The birthday party invitations were sent already with the date, time, and location for the party to be held in a few weeks. I thought, *how could Chrisette's cousins and newly met friends at school attend her birthday party amid social distancing?* This news was disappointing, but we understood why these measures had to be implemented.

As a techie, every Wednesday on Facebook Live, I share marketing strategies to help local businesses grow their reach and revenue as well as retirement readiness strategies. But Wednesday, April 1st, was Chrisette's birthday. Sharing my normal Facebook Live was not on my mind; instead, I decided to do what is normally done for someone's birthday on Facebook. I created a post asking family and friends to wish Chrisette a Happy Birthday. She received around sixty-to-seventy likes and comments. But then, my God-given creativity kicked in. Instead of doing the normal Facebook Live at five PM, I decided to have a Happy Birthday Chrisette Facebook Live! And what a success it was! Instead of sixty-to-seventy people, we had over three hundred people to wish her Happy Birthday and send birthday money as we listened to music, danced, ate cupcakes, and played with balloons live with family and friends. Chrisette said this was the best birthday party ever!

How cool is that? Did that encourage you? Have you taken the time and creativity to bring joy to someone today? That creativity that is lying dormant in you, I speak life to it right now. So, get ready. Find a pen and paper, a quiet place and talk to the creator of the universe – the Almighty God, the God who knows all, sees all and cares. As he reveals to you the thing that he wants you to bring forth and spread from person to person, begin to tell Him thank you. Tell Him how grateful you are that He is a faithful God. Thank him for clarity, 2020 vision and provision to get it done.

You, too, may have felt disappointed about the coronavirus. But rest assured, there is nothing too hard for God. So, be encouraged in the Lord because you were placed in the kingdom for such a time as this. May the Lord bless everything you put your hands to do. Sure, wash your hands, but at the same time, wash your mind of wrong thoughts, doubt, and fear. I pray that the Holy Spirit will empower you to cast down every thought and imagination that tries to exalt itself over God's Holy Word and plan for your life. Know that the hand of the Lord is with you to lead and guide you throughout the process. Thank God for extending your borders and reach while social distancing. Yes, the coronavirus is doing what it does by spreading germs and sickness that leads to death; but I pray that you trust God, tap into your God given creativity, and let the Lord use you to spread joy, hope, and encouragement that leads to life.

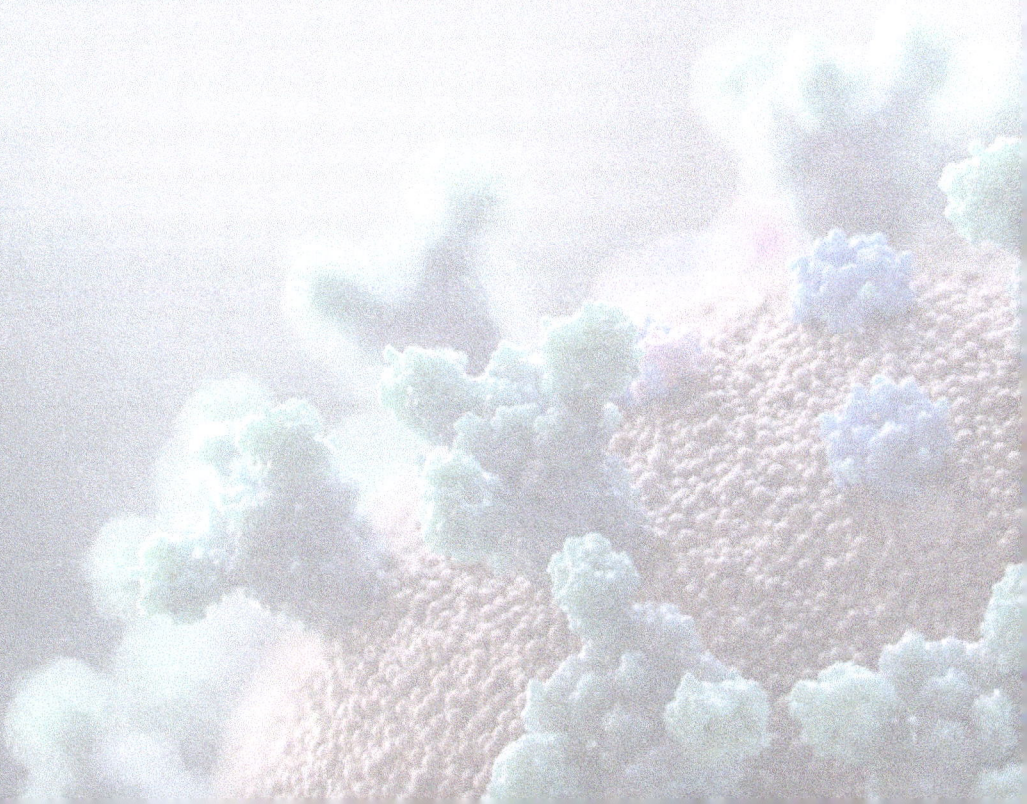

VOLUME II

Confinement Chronicles

How God Got Me Over The Curve

Encouraging Testimonies Birthed from the 2020 Coronavirus Pandemic

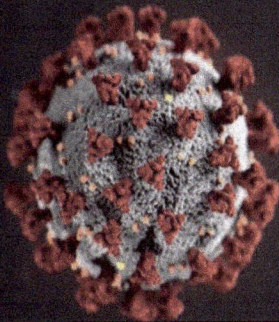

An inspirational audiobook compilation series
Produced by

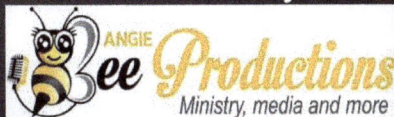

ANGIE Bee Productions
Ministry, media and more

COVID-19 AND LONGING FOR A JOY THAT IS COMPLETE:

Restoring My Joy

Vernessa Blackwell

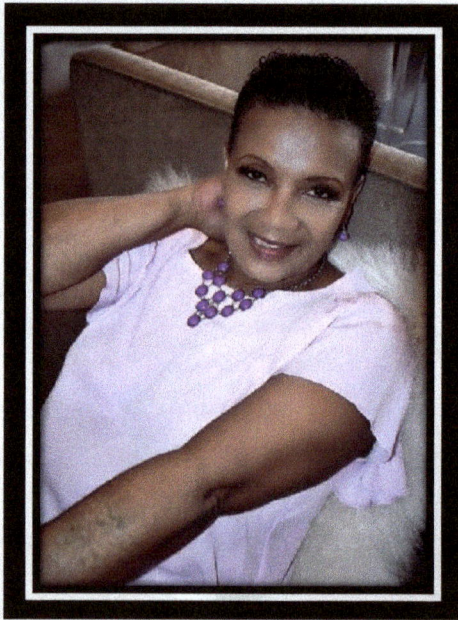

As we navigate the changes that come with COVID-19, recall that times of uncertainty can be stressful ...

We worry about so many things! We want to know: why have we had to suffer the loss of a loved one? Why did our loved one make such a foolish choice? The "why" questions reveal our inner desire to be in control, and when we are not in control, we are filled with worry, grief, and despair.

God gives understanding, but it is a gift to the heart to rest in Him. The good news is that we can learn the things that make for peace. We can learn to pray the

Jesus way. We can cultivate thankfulness that springs from the heart. We can experience peace. He calls us to learn from Him.

Take some time to reflect: how can I keep inspired and restored during uncertain times? Make space for creativity and humor.
Ask, "What calls forth my joy?"

CHANGE US, LORD

I do pray that this unprecedented season and our extra reliance on technology will result in positive change within the body of Christ.

We can start here.

BEGIN TO USE SCRIPTURAL AFFIRMATIONS AND POSITIVE AFFIRMATIONS.

Affirmations are the most encouraging and inspirational words! They are Biblical affirmations that are backed by scripture. They will help you to speak God's Word and believe God's promises for your life! They will help you to stay thankful and appreciate all of your blessings. Affirmations work! The power of affirmations has improved the lives of millions of people! The Bible says that *death and life are in the power of your tongue* (Proverbs 18:21 KJV).

I CHOOSE JOY!!!!!

If you CHANGE your words, you can change your life! Christian affirmations are the most powerful affirmations because you will be speaking God's Word! You will be filled with faith and confidence. God is BIGGER than any challenge you face! Whatever your goals and dreams are, you can do much more WITH GOD than without Him. Jesus said, *With God all things are possible* (Matthew 19:26). You *can do all things through Christ* (Philippians 4:13)! Your life will change on the outside, when you change on the INSIDE. Christian affirmations will help you to replace negative thinking with positive affirmations! Replace worldly thinking with scriptural thinking!

They will motivate you, encourage you, bless you, and build your belief! Jesus said, ...*all things are possible to him that believeth* in Mark 9:23. Next to each affirmation is a Bible verse for further study and context. Regular Bible reading will help you discover God's great plan and purpose for your life. Affirmations are, well, affirming statements that you say out loud to yourself on a regular basis. The goal is to re-program your subconscious mind with positive thoughts so that you can remove any negative thoughts preventing you from pursuing your goals and dreams.

You can write your affirmations in your planner or write them out on index cards and keep them with you in your purse. Whenever you have a few moments to spare, take them out, and read them aloud. I like to say affirmations during my morning routine when I wake up to set the tone for my day.

Affirmations to Release Grief & Restore Joy

With every breath I take, I am thanking God for the joy, restoration, and healing to every cell in my body.

Yes, yes, yes, yes. I am restoring my joy.

I release the grief and know that I will recover from this!

Every part of me is getting the optimum benefit from this planner!

Pure joy might seem like a fleeting emotion, but even if you only feel it for a moment in time, you can hold on to it. You can relish in it.

As a Grief and Joy Restoration Coach, it is my goal to inspire you to find joy in your journey. I am Vernessa Blackwell, the Grief Strategist.

SOME PEOPLE WERE ALREADY LIVING IN A "PANDEMIC"

Evangelist Tahara Lee

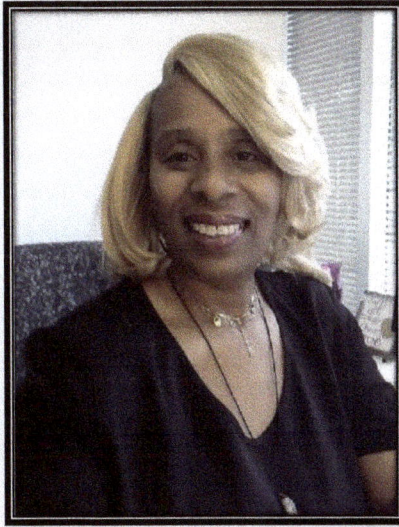

MANY didn't see it; but there were people going through a "pandemic" before corona arrived on the scene. Many people don't see the hurt and pain of others even as they say they are Christians. To be a Christian should demonstrate "Christ-like" actions. Yes – Action; to do.

Romans 10:15 KJV

And how are they to preach unless they are sent? As it is written, "How beautiful are the feet of those who preach the good news!"

1 Corinthians 15:58 KJV

Therefore, my beloved brothers, be steadfast, immovable, always abounding in the work of the Lord, knowing that in the Lord your labor is not in vain.

People go about their everyday lives because they are all right; their family is all right. So, they go through their day not concerned about another person not eating; another family didn't have the money to pay their light bill because they had to pay their car insurance to get the child to the doctor that they need to get through chemo. We are our brother's keeper. To me, this means being there when another has a need. You may not be able to fill the need, but to be there as support can mean the world to a mother that has been crying and only knows words of prayer because they need their child healed. They know the child was a miracle and know God didn't bring the child into the world to take them back. But they need encouraging words to get them through to the healing stage.

So, when the "pandemic" arrived, I believe God was putting everyone on the same playing field, so to speak. There were ones that lost jobs who had worked for years. Now you know the feeling of being unemployed. Not there that is glory in this, but now you can feel how someone was already feeling who was already living through unemployment. To trust in God to provide and not a paycheck. I used to be at a job where the supervisor didn't understand when parents had to take off work to take a child to an appointment; they had to go to the school for a parent-teacher meeting; they had to leave work because their daycare or school called stating the child had a fever, and the parent didn't have a support group to take the child for the day – so, now, that already stretched income is a day shorter.

Since then, (and at that time) she now has a family and has had to walk in the shoes of a parent instead of a single person who doesn't have to be responsible for a family, another person's life; and her outlook at parenting and peoples' requests to leave has taken on a whole new meaning.

There have been mothers, fathers, grandmothers, someone's daughter that died alone in a nursing home or hospital ward because they were estranged from their family. No one came to check on grand mom in the nursing home, and when she went to sleep the night before, they didn't know she wouldn't wake up any more. She died – alone. Where was a loved one that would cry out when they heard the news of her passing but never brought her flowers while she was alive? Yes, people have being living as if we were already in a PANDEMIC.

So, I've written this piece to ask you to continue to be kind to others. We don't know what someone is facing at home. And until you open up and just say "hi" or give someone a kind smile, you can't let God open up in you to know there is a need. I truly thank God for the quiet time. It's that communication with the Father we need to be able to walk in His Righteousness. To have the home in order where God is the head, then Father, then Mother, and they teach together, as one, the children.

When we return to the working world, don't forget the world where God resides, which should be in us. Be kind to one another. See about your neighbor. Forgive if you haven't done so already. Because if this pandemic didn't teach us anything – you really should have learned that LIFE IS SHORT. Live each day like it's your last – as it very well may be.

Be Your Brother's Keeper. Selah ...

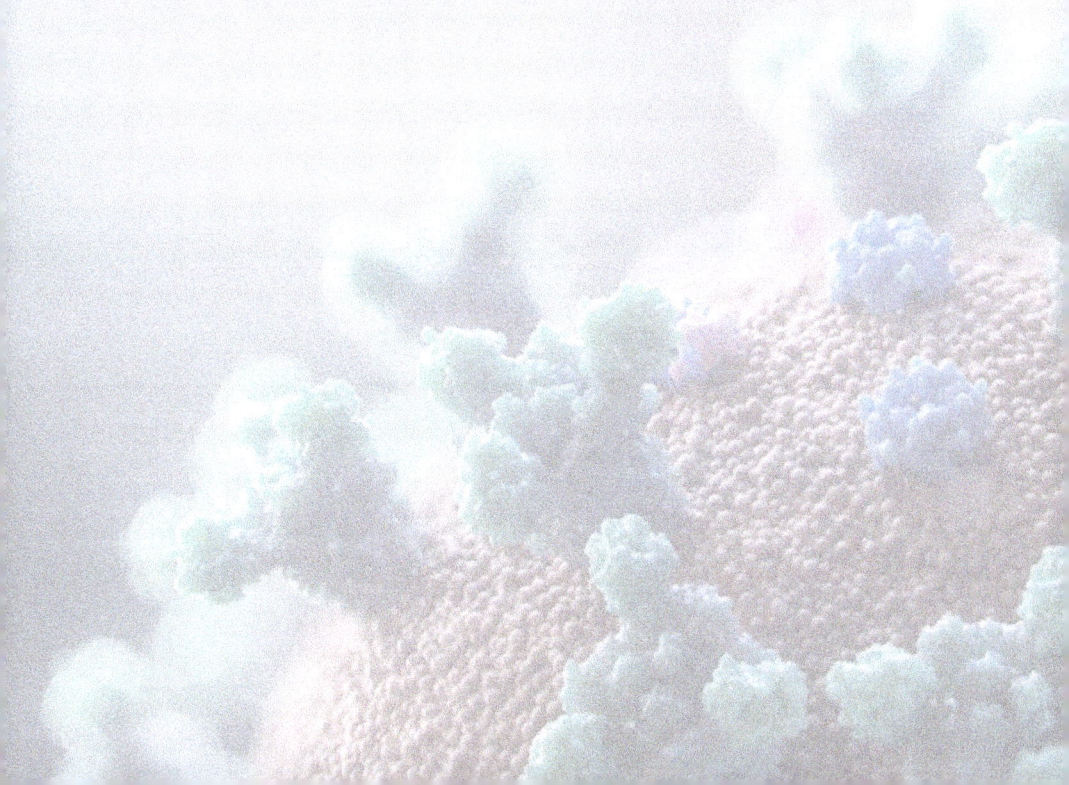

REMEMBER THE LORD

Thaddeus Randolph

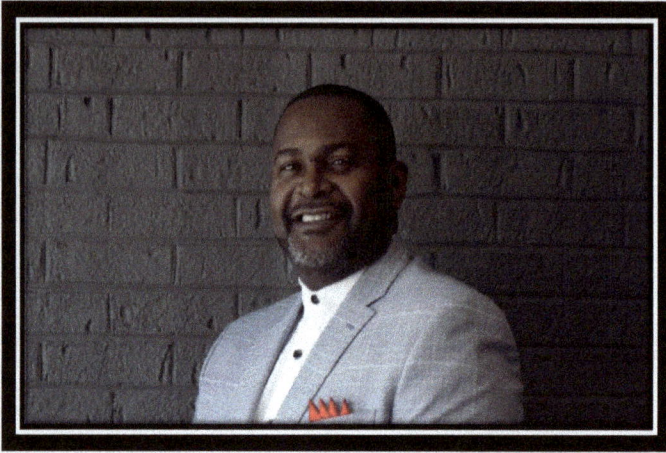

As the seriousness and the urgency of the Coronavirus (COVID-19) pandemic began to come into view, my family and I sat at dinner and talked about how we had never lived through anything like this before. As military veterans, we have both survived deployments to combat zones, lived through the Y2K hype, and lived through the 9/11 tragedy, but this particular crisis is vastly different and presents a potential health threat to us all.

This COVID-19 journey is a new experience for the vast majority of us living today. At the beginning, there were questions concerning the severity of the pandemic and what changes we would have to make as a people and a nation. Once schools and government offices started closing, the present reality of what was occurring across the globe began to settle in. As the virus spread, concerns for personal safety and health, as well as for family and friends heightened. Gathering in churches, schools, theaters, restaurants, and shopping malls created an environment for the virus to spread rapidly. As a man of faith, this outbreak presented an unprecedented challenge to those of us in the faith community.

CONFINEMENT CHRONICLES | 43

How could we maintain our faith and trust in God in the midst of this pandemic?

Daily broadcasts of global, national, and local uncertainty, loss of life, jobs, and failing businesses created atmospheres of panic and fear. As a Ministries Director and Pastoral Care Counselor, attempting to comfort those whose lives had been drastically disrupted presented an unfamiliar challenge for me. Many days, I asked the Lord for wisdom on how to comfort someone whose loved one was severely sick or dying. What do you say to someone who wants to be with their loved one and they're not able to be with them because the fear of spreading the virus is so great? Regardless of how strong your faith is, or even knowing God can heal, does not shield you from the complexities of this pandemic. If you're not careful, the burden to comfort others can wear on you emotionally, spiritually, and physically. Especially, when healing doesn't come and a loved one dies. Even as a person of faith, you may find yourself slipping into moments of depression, doubt, and despair. Let me share some encouragement with you. You are not alone! But, it's in times like this we need to remember that God is there to help.

I'm reminded of a specific time while as a soldier stationed in Germany. My wife and I were enjoying life stationed in Darmstadt, traveling and visiting friends. But then Saddam Hussein invaded Kuwait. Life as we knew it was over. I was reassigned to an Armor Division and deployed in support of Desert Shield/Desert Storm for the Gulf War. All soldiers train in peacetime for what they are called to do in war. There was a lot of uncertainty and apprehension among soldiers about actual military conflict. Specifically, with the threat of chemical warfare and facing Saddam Hussein's vast military forces, we just knew there would be mass casualties. I myself wrestled with uncertainty, and doubt tried to creep into my heart, but I gained encouragement and strength during one of my daily devotions when I read the words of Apostle Paul in 2 Corinthians 12:19 (KJV) *My grace is sufficient for you, for my power is perfected in weakness.* I held onto this scripture throughout my deployment. The outcome of that situation was so different from what we expected. God preserved and kept us through that conflict and gave us a resounding victorious outcome!

There are so many other stories of hope and victory found in scripture where the people of God found themselves in challenging and uncertain situations. There were many times they were outnumbered and surrounded by their enemies, or confronted with sickness and disease. Yet, in all those situations they were encouraged to reflect on and remind themselves of what the Lord had done for them before. One such occasion is found in Psalms 20: 1-9, where the people of God offer up prayer for King David and his army before entering into battle. The people of God are declaring three things - God will defend; God will help; and God will strengthen. In these challenging times, let us declare that God will be our defense, our help, and our strength. May we, like David, remember and proclaim our trust in the Lord.

I encourage you and your families to take time each day to reflect on, remind yourselves of, and remember what the Lord has done, and will continue to do when you put your trust in Him. He is there waiting for us to put our trust wholly and completely in Him. Even in this current crisis, we can be certain that God's grace is sufficient for us.

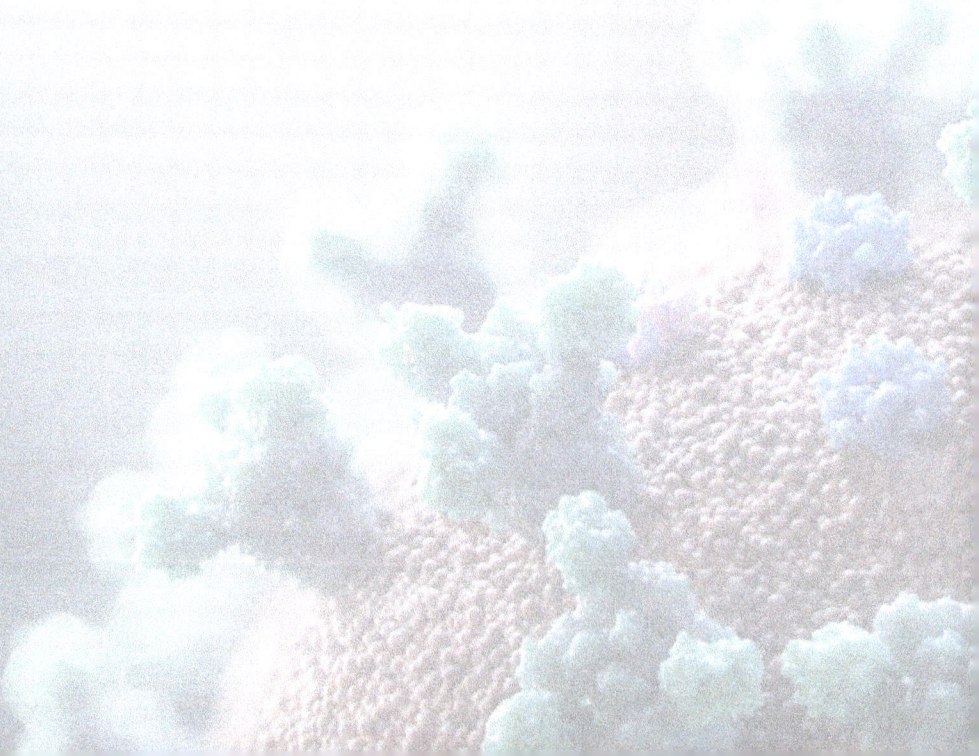

QUARANTINE QUICKIES:

This Way Won't Be Always

Sonya Bennett

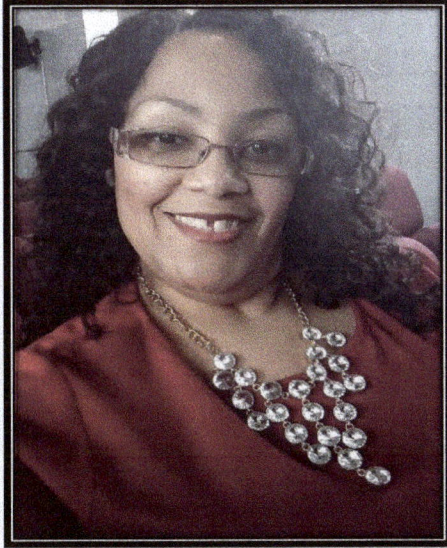

"Idle minds are the devil's workshop" – this older saying still rings true. Here we are: bored in thehouse, in the house bored, and yes, I'm working, my daughter is Google-schooling, but when the day/week/month is over, it's done. How I wish I had gone to one, last movie; they're all closed. Ican still smell the over-priced popcorn that seemed reasonable as we rushed to our seats. I shouldhave gotten a pedicure: where is that pumice stone I haven't used in years; I need it now!

Something else I wish I had gotten just a lil' bit more of: adult, alone time! Being a single parent,I have taken full advantage of that extra time between clocking-out and picking her up from latchkey or an after-school activity: sometimes, that thirty/forty-five minutes give a much-needed "ENTERmission." On rare occasions, I would have some me and he time that gave me a costume-change from Worker to Me to Mommy; it's a way to get over the hump in more ways than one :)

That brings me to my idle-minds reference: being at home all day; you start to investigate other options that you may not have before. Did you know there's a delivery service for EVERYthing: food, clothes, even toilet paper! There are websites for everything from do-it-yourself, do it TO yourself, or find someone. Figured I'd try some out and maybe find a like-minded trapee to chat with and offer a new distraction. I uploaded a few pictures and a short bio that display my wit, humor and desire for temporary, virtual adult companionship. This arrangement seems in high demand; hence, Quarantine Quickies. I found a site that I'll call "You're It" and learned virtual acquainting isn't what it's 'quacked up' to be – everyone wants to exchange numbers or video chat immediately. *Hello?!* Can you ask my name? What happened to courting; we have time! Even real-life flirting can start with subtle glances across the room or non-discreet "stalking" around the grocery store! The worst part is – I've come to realize these buddies won't last. Once the world re-opens, these empty times will be re-filled with normal schedules and these hourly/daily consistent texts will diminish. So, I've closed my heart and opened my mind to short-term exchanges and basement video SEXchanges from Mr. Right Now, and resuming my regularly-scheduled program of believing God for Mr. Right.

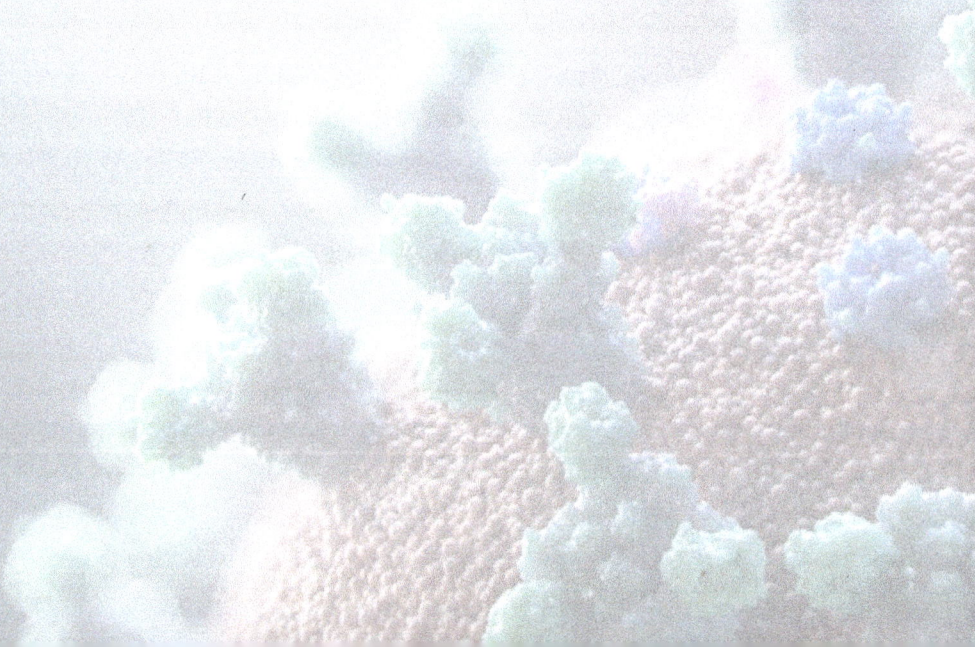

FREE TIME ON MY MIND

Singer and Author BARTEE

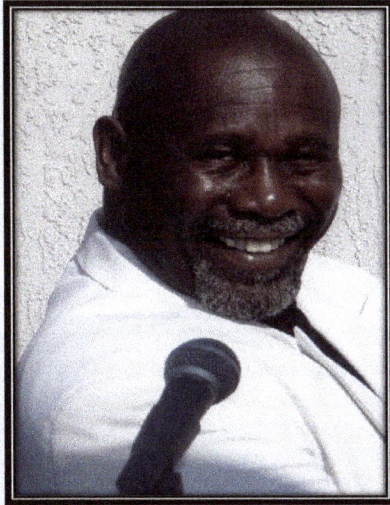

> "*I think of you, sometime, and I want to spend some time with you. We look for love, no time for tears; wasted water's, all that is, and it don't make no flowers grow. Good things might come to those who wait, not for those who wait too late. We got to go for all we know.*"

These lyrics from the Bill Withers song entitled, "*Just the Two of Us*" inspired me to write this chapter.

Spending time with the one you love – Do you want to get away? (Remember that commercial from Southwest Airlines?) Or, is it like having your honeymoon all over again?

During this time of confinement with Corona, it seems like I am cheating on my wife. I stay up late watching TV, and I don't get up in the morning to eat a timely breakfast; I am a bachelor all over again! I sneak around all day with a mask on my face. My wife keeps asking me, "Why you keep washing your hands? Who you been with?!" (LOL)

My wife knows that I am a "One-Woman-Man", so now, it's time for God to remove Corona from my life. "Peace Be Still" (Matthew 8:23).

Coronavirus has changed many people's lives—some for the good, and others beyond comprehension. Traveling by plane, train, bus, and don't forget the cruise ships, is at a standstill. Do you really want to take a chance so soon? Stay prayed-up! Wear your personal protection (mask and gloves, when necessary), and welcome in this new "normal" that God is planning for us!

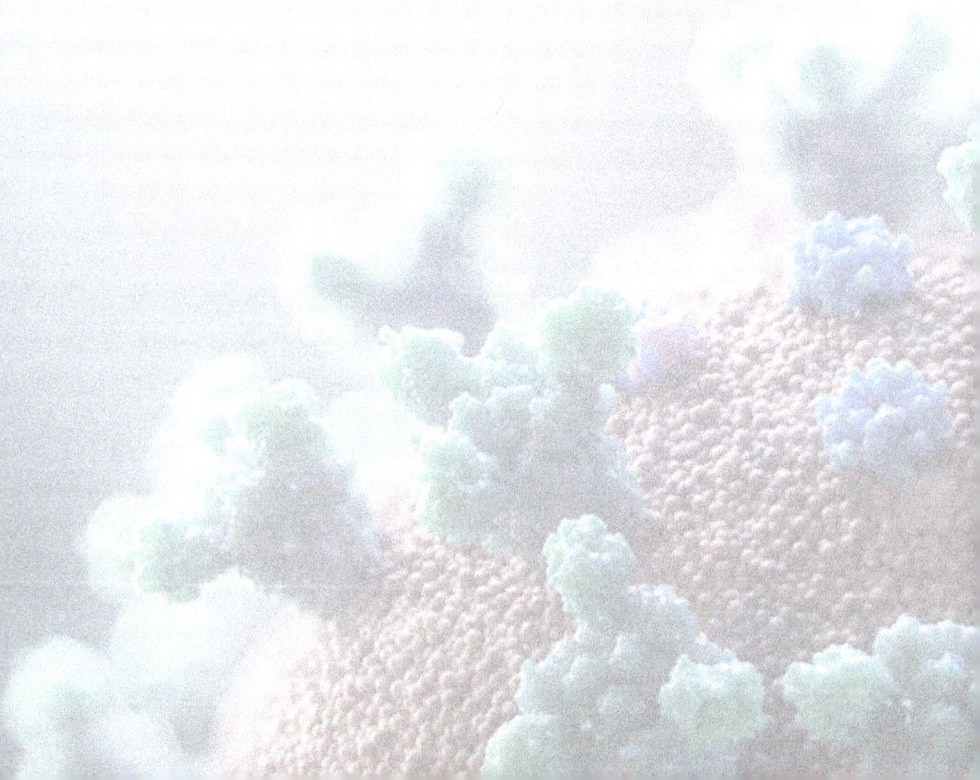

VOLUME III

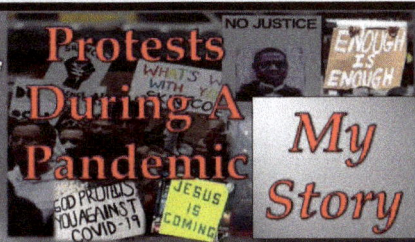

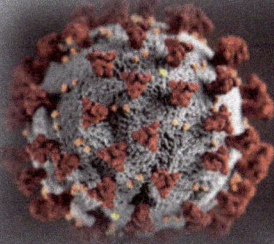

I Can't Breathe!

Volume III of an inspirational
audiobook compilation
series, produced by

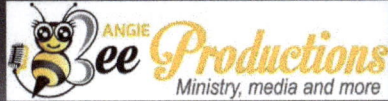

OVERDUE CHANGE IS HERE RIGHT NOW

Theresa Jordan

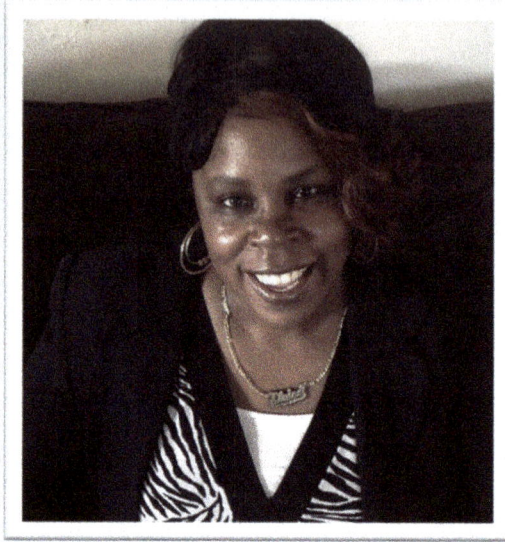

Why are we still encountering these same injustices 401 years later? Why do we have to fight just to be treated like decent human beings? Why do our black men and younger black men have to lower their standards just to make someone else feel like they are more superior? Aren't we living in the year 2020?

Isn't this the United States of America, the land of the free and home of the brave? I thought all men and women were supposed to be treated equally.

Yes, the George Floyd incident was a pivoting point for the Black Lives Matter movement in the United States. But guess what? George Floyd's untimely and unnecessary death on 8/25/2020 – it was the straw that broke the camel's back. Many people still fail to realize it did not just start there. It started with some of the following names: Emmitt Till, Dr. Martin King, Jr., Trayvon Martin,

Michael Brown, Eric Garner, Sandra Bland, Natasha McKenna, Breonna Taylor, Ahmad Aubrey, and Rayshard Brooks.

Haven't we turned our cheeks enough? Haven't we mastered forgiveness by becoming resilient and surpassing past hurts and pain? This should show the world our true worthiness because we have opted to move forward. We have decided to press on to greater heights despite our past circumstances. We are doing this regardless of the repetition of cycles dealing with injustices that have taken place throughout the land. This cycle extends back to our ancestors, our past generations, and now the present and future generations to come.

Well, guess what? Today we decided to collectively take a stand and say, with our words and actions, "Enough is Enough." We will not remain silent anymore, and we will not be complicit to the injustices that are taking place in our world today.

What we are dealing with today reminds me of this scripture, Matthew 20:16 (KJV) *So the last shall be first, and the first last: for many be called, but few chosen.*

Do you know the foundation of the world was created on black men and black women's shoulders? We have stood the test of time because we are destined to be true Kings and Queens. God has given us the knowledge and has purposed in our hearts the need to build and create. Many things were stolen from us, but today we stand here and say: you cannot have our men, and you definitely cannot have our sons; you cannot have our women, and you definitely cannot have our daughters. You have done enough with our past, and we refuse to remain last. Guess what? It was unacceptable in the year 1619 and beyond. And guess what? It is still unacceptable in the year 2020.

Yes, "All Lives Should Matter", so when taking that statement into consideration, remember our worth. We would not have to protest about our rights especially if this was prevalent every day. The protesting should not be taking place during this pandemic, but it is necessary to eliminate overdue injustices. Permanent change is here, and we might not ever experience another explosive movement like this again--at least during our lifetime. History is in the making, and our change has come. This is an enormous movement because it has reached all over the United States and it has reached internationally.

In the famous words of George Floyd's daughter, which were spoken profoundly, "Daddy changed the world." My prayer is that the words that fell off his precious little daughter's lips will reach to our Father above, and her request is answered because of her gigantic faith.

I am grateful that several positive things came forth, and they are still being activated today because of the protesting: Rev. Al Sharpton spoke it best, "If you only knew whose neck you were putting your knee on for 8:46 seconds, you probably would have taken it off George's neck."

You do not have the right to take a father from his daughter or a father from his son. Aren't these the United States of America, where all men and women should be treated equal? These injustices are not telling us the same.

No, this may not take place anymore on our timetable, and it should not have taken place during our ancestors' timetable. The lives we have lost during each cruelty is unacceptable from every prospective. It was not right then, and guess what? It is still not right now. You have picked the wrong generation, because this generation stands firmly upon the shoulders of our dear ancestors.

They also stand on the shoulders of a new generation of young people, who unapologetically are willing to stand up and protest because of injustices. They have decided to treat people the way they expect to be treated regardless of the color of a person's skin. This generation demands to be heard, and they are unstoppable when it comes to doing what is right for their fellow man.

This Black Movement is quite frankly overdue, and despite the pandemic, a tremendous number of great things have come forth. It has stirred up the United States, and it has gone internationally with Black Lives Matter. Artists have come from all over the world to places like Washington, D.C., South Carolina, Hollywood, New Jersey, Cleveland, Ohio, and have written "Black Lives Matter" in the streets. Several countries and nationalities have come together to say, "We are one, and Enough is Enough."

Bubba Wallace has created a movement with NASCAR by having the Confederate flags banned. Statues that supported and perpetrated slavery are being removed, and they are being taking down because they displayed inequality and injustices for the minority race.

My favorite pancake mix and syrup, "Aunt Jemima" is beginning to be removed from shelves. There is a strong possibility that Uncle Ben's rice will eventually be removed from grocery stores due to this incredible movement.

We are living in the times of Sam Cooke's "A Change Is Gonna Come." This song was sung profoundly in the year 1964, and it remains prevalent in the year 2020.

Overdue Change is Here Right Now.

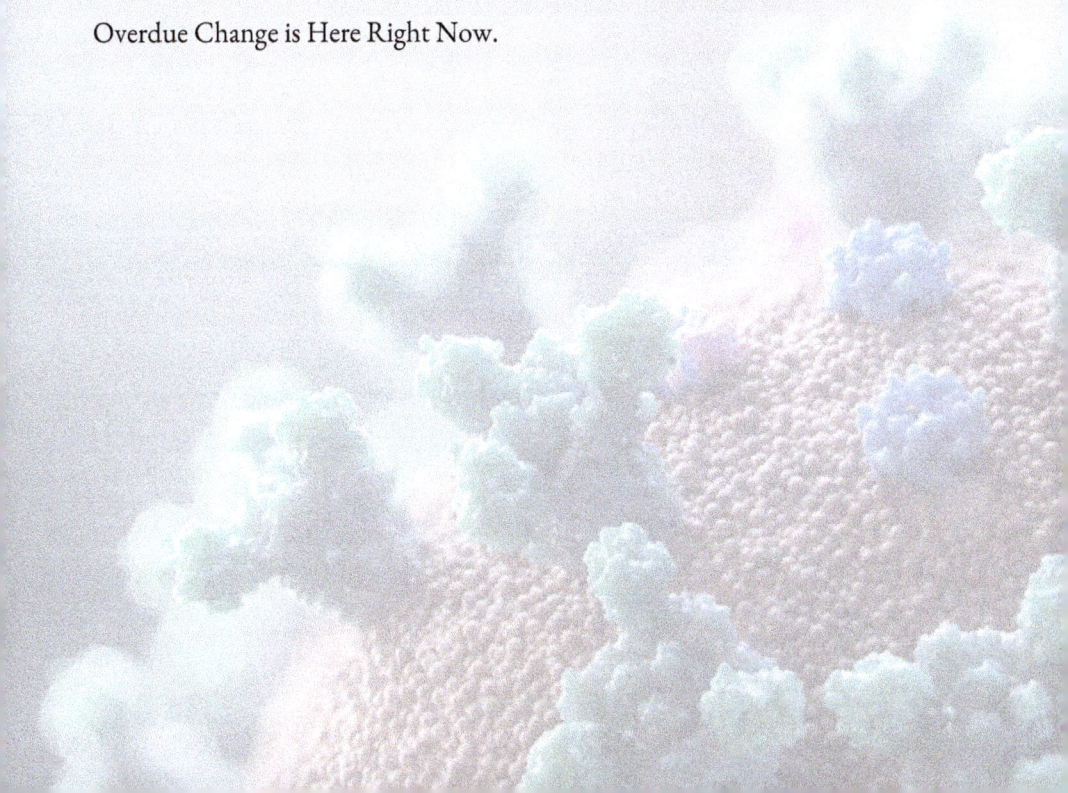

"8:46"

Attorney Regina Nunnally

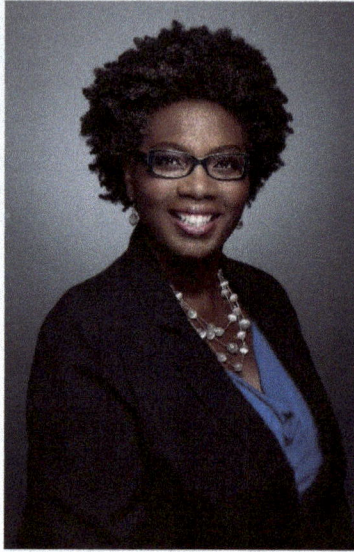

When the year 2020 was anticipated, people saw these numbers as a symbol of clarity of vision. We are heading into a new decade, the Roaring 20s. Then we heard about a virus arising out of China. Then we heard that it was spreading across the world. All of a sudden it was in the United States. How did that bug travel so fast? I mean, was it on a Learjet or something? March 2020, the United States was on lock down. No one could move unless it was totally necessary. Sports, concerts, weddings, graduations ... restaurants, theme parks, vacation plans cancelled. Ugh! I had a trip planned for Cartagena, Colombia. Colombia said, "Nada, chica, no vengas aqui."

Unemployment, cabin fever ... Everyone took to social media for an outlet. Everyone's attention was on the internet. Then suddenly we see a black man shot in the street by a couple of white vigilantes. We hear about a black woman shot to death in her home by police. The proverbial straw that broke the camel's back was a black man strangled to death by a police officer.

I was already feeling some kind of way when I saw Amaud Aubry's death on video. Breonna Taylor being shot eight times while in her underwear, unacceptable. Then I ran across George Floyd's video; I did not want to see it. My mood was already jacked up. The video was going viral, and I could not turn a blind eye. When I saw the video, my gut wrenched! When I saw Amaud's video, I already knew where that was heading. When I heard about Taylor's situation, handwriting on the wall. Finally, George Floyd's video ... due to being knowledgeable, I predicted the reaction, and it came to pass. A certain segment of people like to justify a killing especially when a black man is involved.

However, when I saw a still picture of the officer's eyes, I thought to myself, *He looks demonic.* A morally conscience disconnect. He didn't take that man's cries seriously. People were hollering and trying to intervene; however, the perpetrator had his blue angelic guards to assist. A grown man crying out to his mother who'd been dead two years! I saw probable cause-- a crime being committed.

What happened to 20/20 vision? Where did the ability to see clearly go? When it comes to people in authority and how they conduct themselves, folks become near-sighted, far-sighted, or blind as an armadillo. Another set of numbers had to remove the scales from the eyes of the world. This set of numbers is not scripture or the time on the clock. "8:46," this is how long the officer pressed his knee and full body weight on another human being's neck. "8.46," cutting off his air supply, cutting off his blood circulation. "8.46," causing great bodily harm and death. "8:46," cutting off his generation and cutting him out of his children's lives. He died at the hands of an authority figure that was sworn to protect his constitutional rights.

Protests broke out during a pandemic -- locally, nationally, and worldwide. No one cared about a virus. No one was concerned about social distancing. Although precautions were made, we see now that a man's life is much more precious than who won the World Series. "8:46" exposed the hearts of men, women and children. "8:46" created dialogue that at times was ignored. "8:46" aroused a gentle giant. You see, if I spoke in a calm voice, folks would not listen. If I smiled and said all the right things to be politically correct, you would shrug your shoulders and keep it moving. When I have told you numerous times in a respectful tone that what you are doing is hurting me and offends me, you take it with a grain of salt. But when enough is enough, must I now go "8:46" on you? Louder and a bit petty at times. Cannot get anything done as a dove, got to go bird of prey. Protests and riots occurred. I marched in the rain and spoke my feelings to the crowd. My heart ached. Folks getting tired of being taken for granted. Systemic racism is alive and well. "8:46" was the world's wake-up call to get out of the bed of contentment. "8:46" was the ophthalmologist appointment that adjusted the world's vision to see that black lives always mattered.

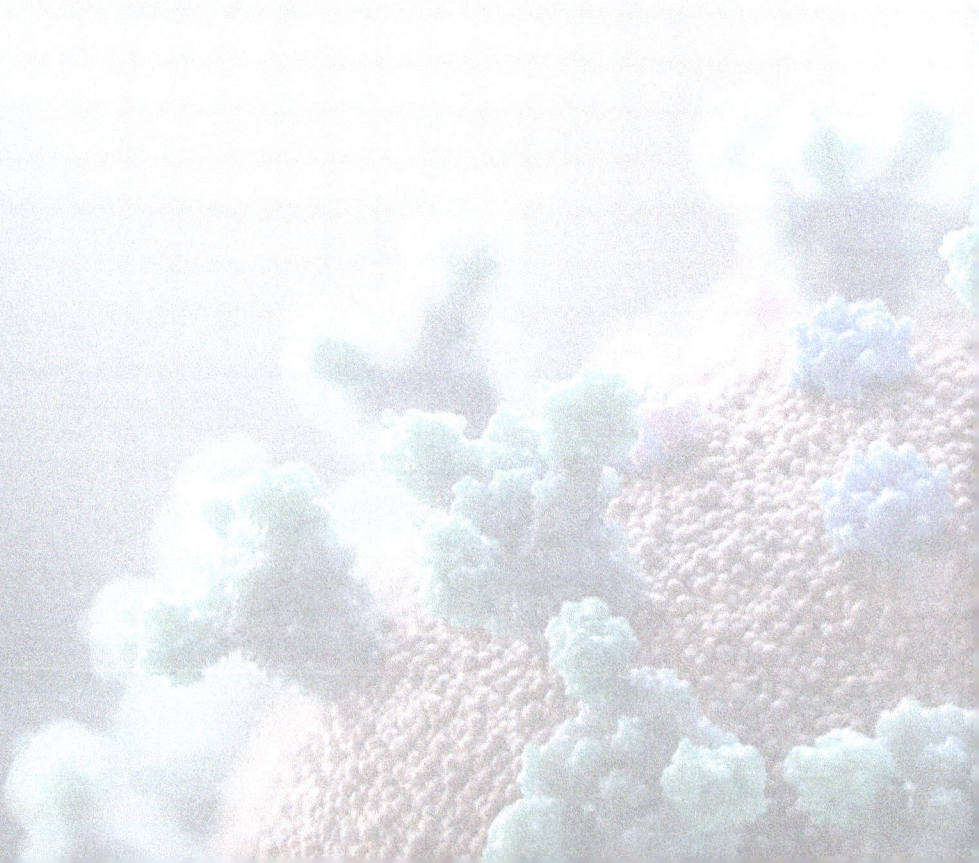

COVID-19 CHRONICLES

Listening to the Angels' Voices and
Being Satisfied with the Creator's Grace

Donna M. Gray-Banks

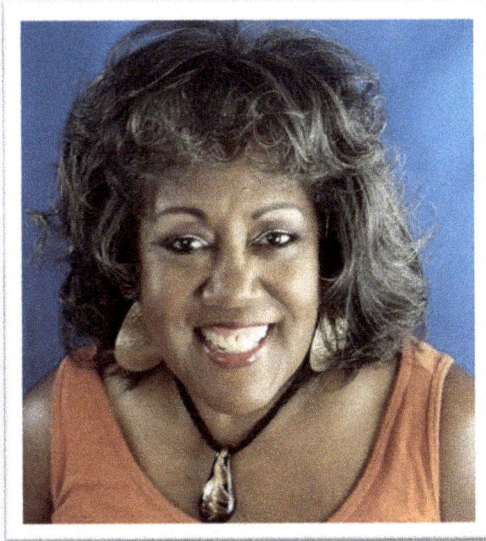

Joel Osteen Quote:
Don't put a question mark where God has put a period.

March 2020

Month 1 - I was so excited about not having to get up every day and put business clothes on to go to meeting after meeting that for the first week, I stayed in my pajamas just because I could.

Week 2 – Still basking in the realization that I did not have to drive anywhere, meet anyone for lunch or dinner, and did not have any client calls. But then on March 2, 2020, I woke up and could not walk – feet swollen, unable to place my feet on the floor. A medical emergency during a pandemic, how was that possible for a person who relishes in being as healthy as possible except for (my) candy crack (which is wintergreen Life Savers®), how could this happen to me? How could I have been told that wearing heels might be the thing of my past and buying expensive tennis shoes that may need to have orthotics placed in them was my new normal? "Don't put a question mark where God has put a period."

Week 3 – Feeling the pinch financially because no one is going to pay you to be in your pajamas all day and reflect on world affairs.

Week 4 – In order to make sure I was secure financially, Zoom became my working partner in the time of COVID-19.

April 2020

Week 1 – Every event that was scheduled for May, June, and most of July had been cancelled, so looking at my calendar with rescheduled or cancelled events became a little depressing. We as adults do not understand how we enjoy human contact until that contact is brought to an abrupt holt and the only communication is the telephone or computer. Then, all of a sudden, there was a toilet paper shortage, and I panicked — for what reason, I do not know. How would I survive? I look back on this day and remember that one of my Angels (my Mother) said to me, "Maria, when the rapture comes, you will not need toilet paper." I cried and remembered that newspaper is also a paper product that could be used, or a washcloth, or paper towel, or wet wipes, or a hundred other things ... 'cause when the rapture comes ... Thanks Mom.

Week 2 – Is makeup really important? While I was one who would not go to the mailbox without lipstick, this pandemic really helped me to realize that people either did not care that I wore makeup or did not want to hurt my feelings and tell me, "Lady, you need to go put on makeup."

Week 3 – Hair and makeup were no longer priorities, but getting in the best physical shape that I could get in considering my age became the battle cry. Up every evening to the park to walk one mile, which I thought was a major accomplishment, then to sit for another hour to bask in the joy of the tremendous exercise I had just done.

Week 4 – Recognizing that a one-mile walk is something you could do around your house. It was important to up the game to two miles at the park.

Week 5 – Starting to count my blessings. I had not missed one F.R.E.S.H. Conversation show which I host every Monday night on Joy 106.3 FM Daytona Beach and wondered if not for the Creator, how did that continue without a hitch during the pandemic. Now we are in July, and we (Terrance Thomas, the engineer) and I have not missed a beat.

May 2020

Week 1 – Civil unrest and rumblings of widespread police brutality: Ahmaud Arbery, Breonna Taylor, George Floyd, and remembering Botham Jean and countless others who have lost their lives due to systemic racism. The numbers are many and the memories are painful and the teapot began to whistle and finally boiled over. No justice, no peace.

Week 2 – Wanting very much to be a part of the protest movements, but knowing that my age would not allow me to be around so many people without maybe subjecting myself to the virus. But then knowing I could advocate online and help others who may need letters written, phone calls made, etc., my advocacy came from my home office.

Week 3 – The revelation, "Don't put a question mark where God has put a period." I have always been the believer that people deserve second and third chances as many do not understand the meaning of friendship and have a hard time grasping even how friendships and relationships develop and survive. But there were those people, places, and situations that I had let linger in my life, that were really not serving any purpose. They were like bookmarks that never moved to the next chapter.

Week 4 – Unrequited love … "Don't put a question mark where God has put a period." Upping the health game by taking the walking to three miles, helps to not focus on unrequited love.

June 2020

Week 1 – Remembering your gift and talents. Writing my fourth novel has become my true obsession. Having the title "Author" is so important to me. The ability to weave a tale that is believable, sexy, intriguing, and timeless is a true gift, and I will never take it for granted.

Week 2 – My passion for literacy -- "Literacy is a Legacy" – overwhelms me, and I begin to formulate plan A, B, and C in order to have a successful F.R.E.S.H. Book Festival in January 2021.

Week 3 – The elimination of toxic people and behaviors that have for too long become a habit that needed to be broken. Missing my family, mother, father, nephew, lover, who have all transitioned; and, missing my son who has ventured into manhood, making his own mistakes and doing it his way. My greatest accomplishment – having the small part in developing his character and knowing that he is a wonderful man and a great citizen who will make an awesome father one day.

Week 4 – Glowing in the knowledge that everything must change and that I may live to see a world where we will finally have a jury of our peers, that black and brown men and women will finally get some respect when it comes to just being, and that the world finally understands that by any means necessary – a change is going to come.

Why Did You Decide to Be A Part of This Project?

Chronicling one's feelings is not something I do regularly as I am usually the one listening to how someone else feels about a situation. I want to thank Evangelist Angie BEE as I did not realize I had so much to say about my journey during these last three months. I am honored she has given me the ability to have writing therapy which I did not know I needed, but truly I did.

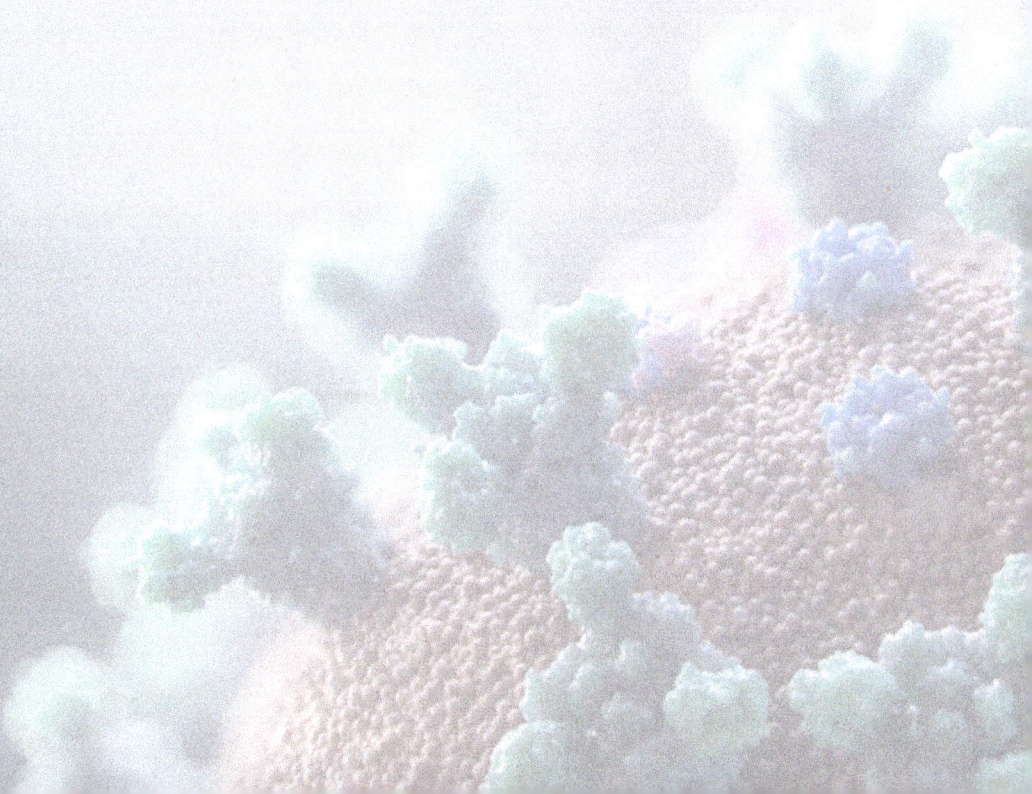

WHO SAID THAT THE REVOLUTION WON'T BE TELEVISED?

Bartee

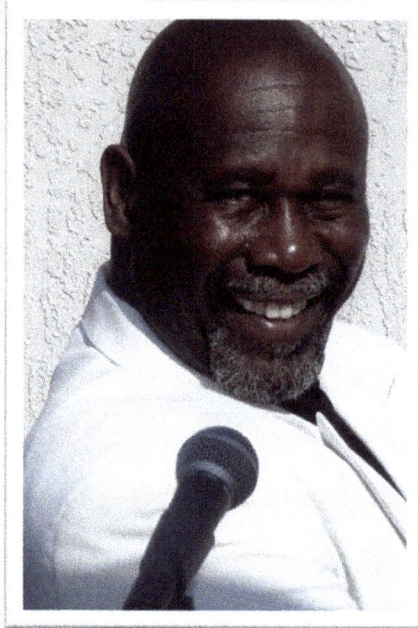

As we prepare ourselves for change, we must understand that accepting crumbs from the "Master's Table" has been given to us, starting with chitterlings. This is the first time that our protests have been shared around the world; and as we continue towards our struggle for "Black Lives Matter", we say to all, "Red, White, and Blue – ALL LIVES MATTER!"

If you have not yet registered to vote, please do so today! If you know a young person that has not yet registered, take them, and introduce them to the options that they will be presented with, on election day.

Stand up, and be counted - VOTE!

Thanks for all those who have laid their lives down, so that we may walk across their bodies saying, "We Shall Overcome, Someday."

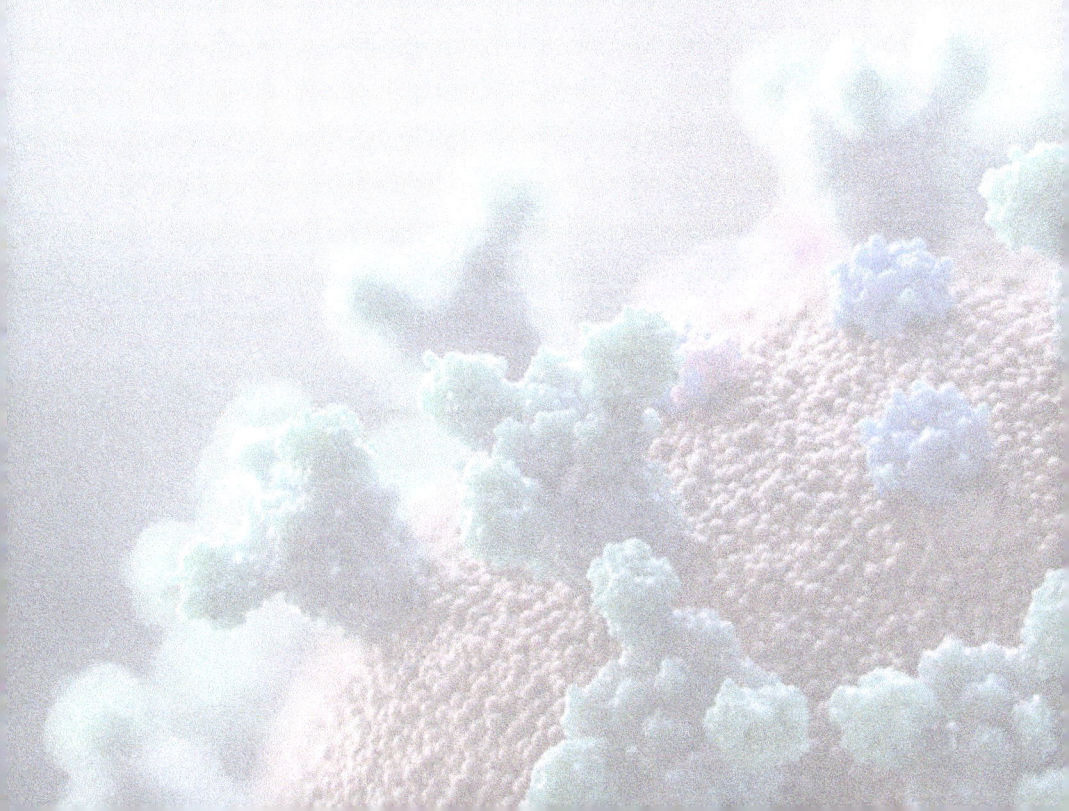

VOLUME IV

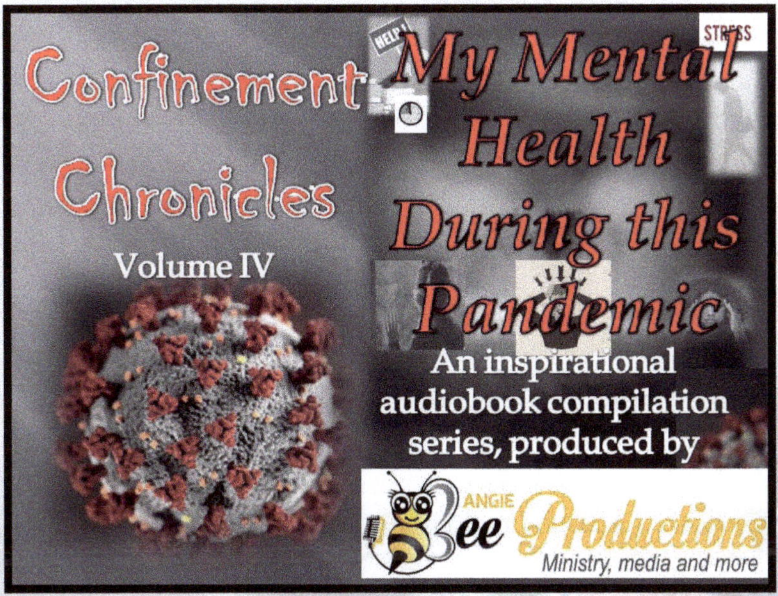
HELP!
STRESS
Confinement Chronicles
Volume IV
My Mental Health During this Pandemic
An inspirational audiobook compilation series, produced by
ANGIE Bee Productions
Ministry, media and more

From Angie BEE

We have arrived at Volume IV, and we are addressing the topic of Mental Health. The month of July is considered Minority Mental Health Awareness Month, yet mental illness does not discriminate due to race, creed, gender or economic status. It attacks the younger and the older, those in good health and those in grief; and if we continue to sit closed-mouthed to the symptoms and solutions, our families will continue to suffer – in silence.

I am grateful for those who God has placed in my life that continue to help me manage the symptoms of my mental illness. I thank God for the prescription medication that I take daily, and I thank Him for the counselors that have provided me with coping mechanisms over the years. As I continue to live with major depression disorder, generalized anxiety disorder, and post-traumatic stress disorder, I strive to share my story with others – to help educate them. Now, as the pandemic rages through our lives and our families, others are experiencing symptoms and they don't recognize them ... they feel lost and confused. It is my prayer that this audiobook will help them to realize that they are not alone, and lead them to seek the help that they need. Share this with others!

And now, for our first contribution...

MENTAL HEALTH THROUGH THE PANDEMIC

Christopher "Swan" Swansburg

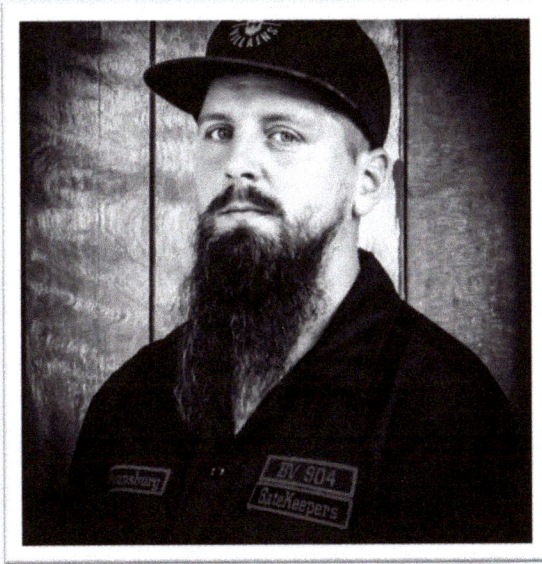

Through the outbreak of COVID-19, we as a nation have had struggles. Our government ignores the experts. Our jobs are looking for loopholes to stay open as essential jobs. Our work hours are reduced. Millions become unemployed. Toilet paper is sold out across the country. Many states reopen too quickly. Protests erupt over police brutality from multiple cases during the pandemic. All while being told "this is the new normal."

As a veteran of the United States Army, having served in Afghanistan, what I see today on the news saddens me. Seeing friends on social media posting how they have lost loved ones due to the virus. Seeing fellow veterans protesting police brutality with signs reading, "I have served my country, I have deployed to war, I retired, and NOW I have to worry about being killed walking to the store because my skin is Brown? This is not the country I served to protect! WE NEED CHANGE NOW!"

The world we live in today does a great job of dividing us. Yet, so many people have come together to help each other. So many people have started to have the discussions needed to help with change. All while living the new normal, wearing masks, social distancing, doing all we can to combat a virus. The virus that shut down the entire world for most people. But what effect does all that is going on in the world have on our mental health? I can only speak to my own mental health and how I have come to cope with the new normal.

Having been to war, I have seen many things most people only see in movies. I have seen injuries that make people squeamish. I have seen such poverty in villages, that once we arrived, even our medical knowledge could not help with the amount of disease that had spread. Yet, I did my job; I came home; I saw a professional therapist for four years to overcome the strain on my mental health. Through those four years of talking to a therapist, I learned techniques that worked for me specifically, to overcome a mental breakdown in today's world. I learned that to clear my mind of negative thoughts, bad news, or simple depression, I tend to focus on work and staying active.

Now, here we are in a pandemic. My job reduces my hours, which means I spend more time at home. My fiancée wishes she could stay home to avoid the virus. I wish I could take a small vacation with my lovely fiancée to help calm her down and clear her head, but the country is closed. The state is closed. So, since I now have more time, I find odd jobs in the house to stay busy and keep my mental health clear and healthy. I start building shelves; I maintain the garden on the patio; I start fixing the minor issues on the cars. I do any and every small job you can think of to stay busy while not at work.

Luckily, I am a member of a brotherhood called The Bearded Villains. My local chapter, here in Jacksonville, has a group chat where we all talk and encourage one another. During this pandemic, we have done a few meetings, charity events, even a day at the beach cleaning up trash to help the environment. This amazing group of men is constantly in communication, working on our next charity event. We are always working on ways to help our local community, from feeding the homeless to cleaning the city streets and beaches. Anything we can do to help our community while keeping ourselves busy during this pandemic.

Now here we are six months into the pandemic, and I am writing my 1st part of a book in my life. I am doing all I can to stay busy. But I have not even started to mention where most of my actual stress is coming from. My stress is not from work; it is not even from fear of the virus. My stress is from planning a wedding for October 2020, with the hopes that this pandemic will die down and allow me and my fiancée to continue with our wedding. A wedding that has so much money already invested, invites and RSVPs sent out, decorations and outfits purchased. How will this pandemic affect our wedding? Will we still be able to use our venue? Will we be forced to reduce our guest list due to limits on those who can attend?

With the stress of a wedding being planned, working during a pandemic, and trying to keep myself healthy to avoid spreading the virus to my family, the strain on my mental health is there; however, through the techniques taught to me years ago, I can manage my mental health and remain calm for those who seek an ear to vent to or guidance on how they should proceed. I am lucky and blessed to have my amazing fiancée, as I keep her mind clear and happy, ensuring her mental health is good; she does the same for me. We have serious discussions nightly about how our days went, what issues we had, what joys we had. We then discuss wedding planning together, between what vendors we spoke to, how they want to proceed. Finally, we discuss our future, having conversations about politics, how we want to raise our children, will we vaccinate our kids, will we give them money when they lose a tooth or do their chores. My fiancée and I ensure we end our nights on good notes before we retire for the day to our bed, to ensure no negative thoughts are in our minds as we sleep. That is how I have handled my mental health through the pandemic. How have you?

THE JOY OF THE LORD IS MY STRENGTH

Theresa Jordan

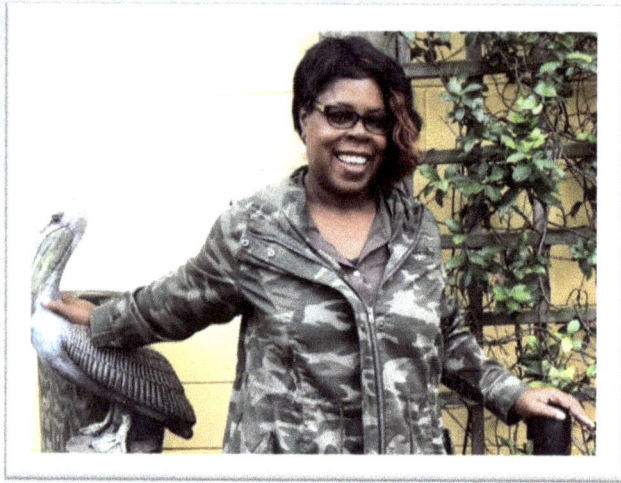

"My mental health during COVID-19?" Let me tell you that I am grateful that I know, and I have King Jesus in my life. Our church would often sing a song called, "In A Time Like This I Need the Lord to Help Me." I believe it was sung by Isaac Douglas & Savannah Mass Choir in 1981. I have been pulling on everything that has been embedded in me: for example, the Word of God, past lessons taught by my Pastor Larry D. Chavers, Sr., and Evangelist Althea R. Chavers, listening to audiobooks such as, *Confinement Chronicles* by the fabulous and amazing, Angie BEE. I have also learned in this season that God is investing in me, and He is allowing me to press pass my comfort zone. He is taking me to places that I would have never imagined or quite frankly thought were possible.

This month marks four months that we have been dealing with COVID-19, and many lives have been lost and changed during this pandemic. I do not want to disregard or not acknowledge the families that have lost loved ones due to the coronavirus; especially, with numbers escalating every day at an alarming rate. When I reviewed it last, it was greater than 130,000 in the United States. I am reminded during this time that there are some husbands that did not have the opportunity to say goodbye to their wives or their children. There are some wives that did not have an opportunity to say goodbye to their husbands or their children. I can recall several years ago, a seasoned young lady approached me during my banking days, and she requested for me to remember to pray for our world. I did not realize the severity of her petition; however, it became more prevalent to me during the coronavirus. Now, do not get me wrong, I have always prayed for our world, but it has escalated over the past four months, because I know people are heavily relying on my prayers to receive their breakthroughs. I am a witness that prayer changes things, and that may be the only antidote to bring that man, woman, boy or girl out of their current circumstances.

There is a song called, "Somebody Prayed for Me" ... they had me on their minds, and they took the time to pray for me. I know that someone is totally relying on that prayer no matter where they are. That person could be here in the United States, or internationally, and that person could be our next-door neighbor. It could also be someone in our family encountering this unimaginable virus. The world needs our prayers right now, besides someone is totally relying on them. Our prayers could change the entire universe, and our prayers do not cost you or me anything. One thing is certain about this virus is it has no respect of persons. In other words, it does not care if you have money, and it does not care if you do not have money. It does not care if you are famous, and it does not care if you are infamous. Coronavirus does not discriminate at all, not even for a moment. Fortunately, New York records have decreased enormously, but I also know it takes an excellent leader. I commend the Governor of New York, Andrew Cuomo, for doing a remarkable job to decrease the number of cases they were experiencing in the beginning.

I believe we can learn substantially from New York and other places that have deescalated the numbers of deaths from here and abroad. What has been keeping me is knowing Proverbs 3:5-6 says, *Trust the Lord with all thine heart,*

Theresa, *and lean not to your own understanding.* Verse 6 continues, *In all your ways,* Theresa, *acknowledge Him and He shall direct your paths.* Now, I have personalized it myself by inserting my name, and of course, you are more than welcome to do the same. In other words, I am learning enormous things through YouTube, Zoom; and I am learning how to start pampering myself more frequently. I am working toward eating healthier foods, because at the beginning of the year I promised myself that I wanted to lose weight. My plan is to accomplish this by November 2020 in honor of my mother not being here. My mother passed due to heart disease, and that is a promise that I have made to myself that I will do better. I have had my moments, especially since we are spending an insurmountable amount of time at home due to the virus.

Someone once told me, "If you want something different you must do something different." Therefore, I am making myself accountable by working out either on my treadmill or stabilized bicycle. It has been mentioned, "If you repetitively do something more than twenty-one days, then it becomes a new habit for you." With that being said, I am reprogramming myself to eating earlier than 6:00 PM, and I am focusing on working out more often. This has helped me mentally, physically, and spiritually because I have gained a new perspective on life.

I am blessed to be part of a spectacular group of authors in *Confinement Chronicles,* and I didn't realize that in this season, God is enlarging my territory. I am grateful that in this season He thought enough of me, and I do believe deep inside my heart, Theresa, you have not seen anything yet because the best is yet to come. In this season, I am learning to be grateful about everything because the scripture says, *In everything give thanks: for this is the will of God in Christ Jesus concerning you.* (1 Thessalonians 5:18)

It is funny because when I was in banking, a client of mine mentioned to me, "Theresa, you are never going to stop going to school," and she mentioned that I would never stop learning new things. When she made that statement, I just laughed and laughed, because I was not seeing what she was seeing for me; however, the good Lord allowed her to see it beforehand because He knew it would be manifested into my life. With that being said, I would like to express my gratitude to Angie BEE and Bartee for always pulling the best out of each of us, even when we did not see it for ourselves. You push every one of us to our fullest potential and our God-given destiny. You could have not listened when the Lord whispered into your ears that *Confinement Chronicles* would need more than sixty minutes, and it would grow substantially in this season and beyond. Angie BEE reminds me of the Clark Sisters' mother, Dr. Mattie Moss Clark; she was able to push each of her daughters into their fullest purpose and destiny, which caused each of them to reach their fullest potential. They could not see it for themselves, but she visualized it beforehand, and the good Lord allowed everything she saw to materialize into their lives. It was by her faith that her daughters surpassed even their own imaginations. Dr. Mattie Moss Clark did an exceptional job, and it is phenomenal how she envisioned everything long before her daughters did, and then they conceived it and envisioned it for themselves.

This is a new season, and I plan to embark upon everything that my heavenly father above has set aside for me. I do not want to miss anything looking to the left, and I do not want miss anything looking to the right. I just want to be in right position to receive everything that He has in store for me. I declare and decree, "This is my season, and this is my time!"

Thank you, Jesus, for this remarkable season because everything is turning around for me, and I thank Vashawn Mitchell for reminding us during this season everything is turning around for you, and everything is turning around for me. I am grateful despite everything happening around us in the year 2020, I can say, "The Joy of the Lord is My Strength."

POEM

"Delivered, Healed, Set Free from the Inside Me"

Ivy Sebastien

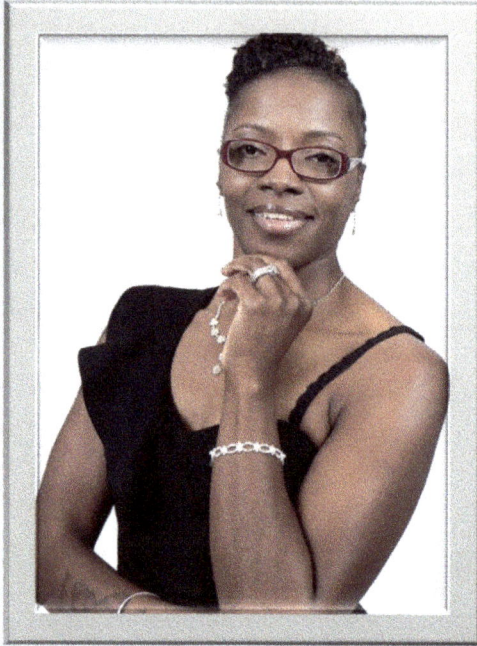

The it in me, captured, tortured traumatized & held in bondage,
Not yet free, from Genesis, my beginning, born in sin
Not knowing who I was within
From the dust of the earth, ABBA father is the essence of a new birth
Oh but the it in me never the less would let me exodus
But from the beginning I knew I was Leviticus the called
I was in numbers my wilderness, it was
Yeshua who came to recompense, to repair to reward
I did not know or understand this Bible called the sword
Yeshua paid the price as my reward for the it in me
He prepared the way he came to deliver and set free
ABBA because of your Shekinah Glory I am able to tell my story of the it in me

The lies, deceit, fornication, lust the darkness that was powers to be

Oh father what I did was due to the it in me but Abba you gave me

The Deuteronomy the instructions, no I did not take heed of the instructions

You gave for me wow you call me Joshua your salvation, I see the compilation

Galatians 5:22-23 of peace, joy, love, meekness, long suffering, faith, gentleness, goodness &

temperance of this one true worshipper, yes the laborer, worker, toiler & servant to you

My almighty king, Abba you took the pain, hurt, resentment, insecurity, rejection, lust & lies

Out of the it in me My word my word it is the Judges yes deliverer, defender, savior, protector,

teacher, leader, vindicator that be as I sit and ponder over my life abba you gave the law

The grace & mercy Yeshua is one who gave his life on Calvary

For the it that was in me

No longer in bondage, slaved, sinful, in tangled with the it in me

From Genesis to Revelations you gave the instructions, the law,

You gave Yeshua who came to fulfill the law, not change one jot or tittle

I walked through it, read it, trusted it you see

My sword & peace, Thank you, Yeshua, Thank you

For all the work you you fixed in me

To save & deliver me from the people and the it in me

HURT PEOPLE, HELP PEOPLE!

Monique Chandler

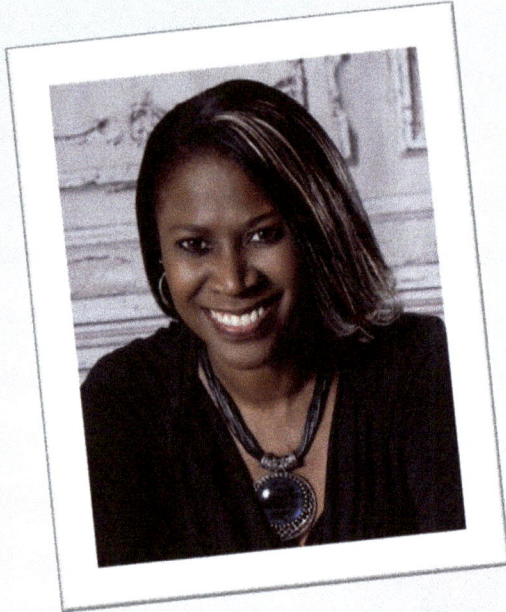

Y ou may call him Officer Jekyll, but I now call him Mr. Hyde, and for very clear and obvious reasons. Strange thing about a pandemic, some of us have nothing on our hands but time. When all the busyness of my life came to a screeching halt, I was forced to deal with "the us" that we once were. The world sees you, Mr. Hyde, as such a loving person. But in our world, you were killing me with your words and lack of action. The intentional hurt and words you utter do matter. Being a Black woman in America, I have become accustomed to certain treatment, but home is the one place where I should be able to have peace. As an officer of the law, you tell your recruits that they have the ability to strip people of their humanity. Did you ever stop to consider how you were stripping me of mine?

Why did you feel the need to share my perceived faults with everyone except me? Why did you take the time to learn my triggers, only to use them against me to justify your actions? The sabotage to our relationship was intentional and left me numb. All I wanted to do was love you in the way that I, too, wanted to be loved.

It has been two years since you walked me through the darkest season of my life. You made, and still make, light of your wrongdoings and intentional abuse. You moved on rather quickly because you were full of crap from the start. For months, I've been sleeping on me, forced to deal with the burden of healing from all the drama and stress you put me through. Your preference was for me to move on, and I have. You see, I have a tele-therapist that I choose to maximize for my growth. Making that choice was not optional for me, it was mandatory because I made it that way ... for me!

It is true that hurt people hurt people, but it is also true that people who have allowed themselves to be helped can also help people. I tried (to help you), but until you feel the need to seek help and get help, you will never be healed and your pattern of abuse will continue. Suffering in silence and refusing to deal with your issues is your choice because help is available, and you have unrestricted access to it.

Accepting the truth of us is hard, but necessary. It only took a few minutes' worth of conversation for me to break down and cry for twenty-four hours straight. Every emotion I ever suppressed while attempting to hold on to the fallacy of our relationship bubbled up to the surface. I was hurt, I was angry, I was sad, and I was frustrated. But on the other side, I found my happy, my peace. I'm up now! I'm awake! I'm all the way awake! Yes! As your cousins would say, "I'm Woke!" And I plan to #StayWoke! I wish you no harm as you continue on life's journey. Know that karma is real. Know that karma has no expiration date. You tried to kill my spirit. You tried to smother my ambition. You even tried to strangle my drive, but I was able to get your knee off my neck. Thank goodness I was able to catch my breath, exhale, shake off the dust, and push forward.

Strange thing about a pandemic, some of us have nothing on our hands but time. I am woke now. I no longer go around putting out fires for people who are addicted to the flames. I sure hope you haven't put your knee on anyone else's neck.

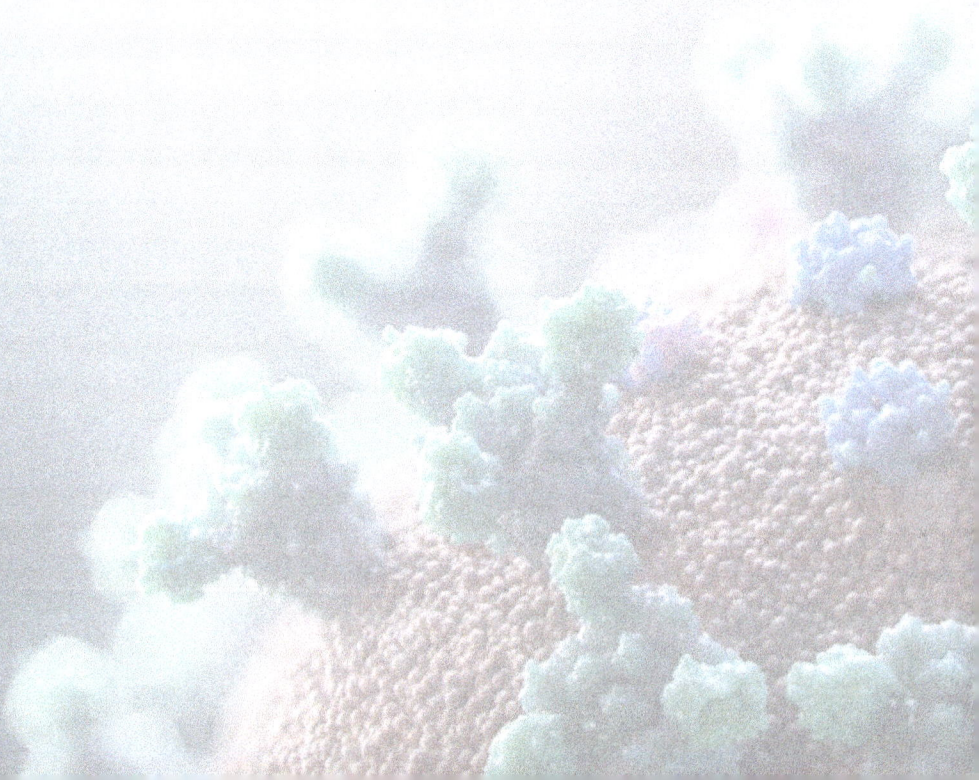

3-1-3 MENTALITY

Sonya Bennett

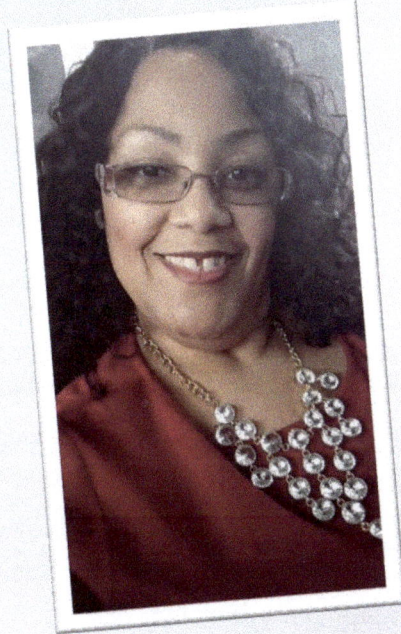

March 13th – "3-1-3": the day my world changed and our thoughts about 'normal' will never be the same.

March 12th: mumbling about schools closing, office positions transferring to work-at-home havens, delivery services booming as our Mayor – affectionately dubbed "Big Gretch" – passes an Executive Order to stay-home, stay-safe. I've never wanted to go out and play so much in my life! The hassle to mask up and glove up wasn't so bad in those end-of-winter months; hell, those kept my face and hands warm. March in Michigan is still very cold; ask the Snowbirds who migrate to Florida every year.

Then, the reality of the 3-1-3 Mentality began to expand: carry hand sanitizer, spray disinfectant, "Hey! Leave those shoes at the door, throw your clothes in the hamper and get in the shower" – my battle cry to my then seven-year-old who was my constant shadow since there is no school, and there are no activities (like movies), no playdates – not even a church service. How frustrating for her and me as the days inch by, and we muddle through virtual school, online and telephonic work duties and constant togetherness. Then it hit me: how will I celebrate her upcoming 8th birthday? We can't go to the arcade-with-the-mouse-character, we can't even have an ice cream cake made; everything is closed.

That 3-1-3 Mentality: it all started March 13th, when my world changed.

I, literally, was in tears as I realized this new "virtual birthday party" is my only option. My sister suggested an Amazon Wish List, online cash-sending option, and maybe, a virtual party would be in order. Being an only child, I have endeavored to create a birthday celebration every year of her young life; even if it was just family. I wanted her to know that birthdays are not promised: 2020 has definitely underscored that truth. I urgently reached out to her teacher to ask if she could contact as many classmates as possible to get together virtually on her birthday. I also scheduled a family virtual party that included church friends and unexpected guests. Tears of joy all around, as heads 'Zoomed' in and out saying "Happy Birthday" Our special 'Angel' hand-delivered homemade cupcakes and for a couple of hours, the world made sense again.

The 3-1-3 Mentality: March 13th, the day my world changed.

It Is Well With My Soul

Marcus Latimer

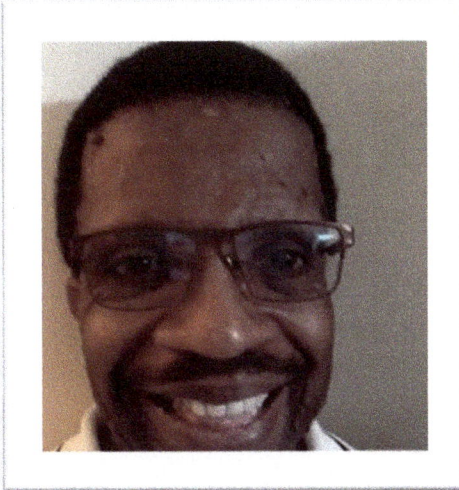

On April 22nd, one week after being admitted to the hospital during the pandemic, my father passed away of bile duct cancer, which we didn't know he had. Not being able to visit him was hard on me and my mom, but the Lord still answered my prayer after receiving the news from the doctors. I prayed, "Lord, if you're going to take him, please wait till morning"(my brother passed at about 2am on Sept 20th 2018); my request was honored.

We lost several family members, friends, and church members to the VIRUS. The hardest part was not being able to meet and console each other in-person. The Lord provided me with female friends who had lost loved ones prior to and during the pandemic. They each gave me powerful words of encouragement! (I guess God used women to say if they can get through this, so can you!) He also led me to many scriptures like 27th Psalm (KJV), Psalm 118: 24 (KJV), and Isaiah 40:31 (KJV).

Growing up in the choirs of Hartford Memorial Baptist Church, it was music that calmed my spirit the most. Songs like "The Lord Is My Light" by the New Jerusalem Choir of Flint Michigan; Reverend Charles Nicks and the St. James Choir songs "I Really Love the Lord", "Oh Give Thanks", and "I Can Depend on God"; James Cleveland's "God Is", "Down Through the Years", and "Through It All" are some of the songs that came to me. It's like I heard someone say, "If It's In You, When You Need It, It Will Come Out of You!"

The powerful hymns that also brought comfort were "Great Is Thy Faithfulness", "Amazing Grace", "Blessed Assurance" and "It Is Well With My Soul" to name a few.

The Lord has used, and is still using, these things to help me get through. Donald Lawrence and the Tri-City Singers song titled: "The Best Is Yet to Come" is what I use on my texts and email communications.

"Have A Great Life! The Best Is Yet to Come!"
Marcus Latimer

And now, for our final contribution...

YOUR HARVEST YEAR – DOUBLE IS YOUR PORTION!

Dr. April L. Johnson

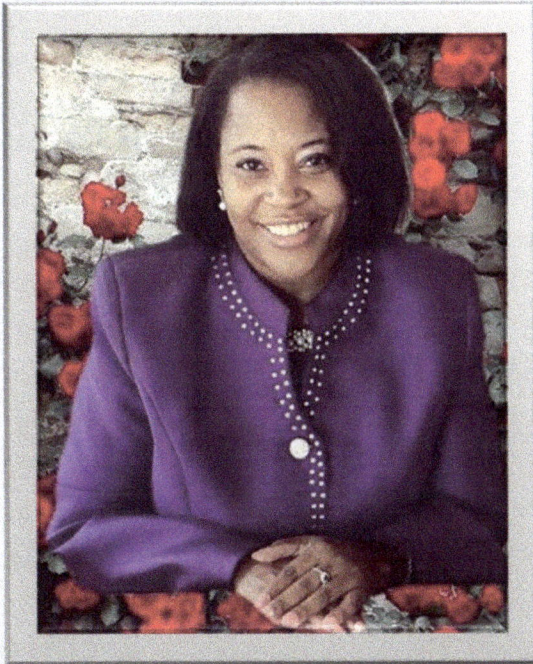

A s I was reflecting in meditation during this unprecedented time of the Coronavirus pandemic, my heart was heavy for those that lost lives in their family, and I was celebrating the success stories, as well, for the survivors of the disease. I was seeking direction for the upcoming months as the first few months of 2020 have been explosive and appearing contrary to the declarations made at watch night services and yearly resolutions. Some have also shared that 2020 will be a year of clear vision or perfect vision, which I don't doubt because the Lord speaks to manifest himself to us in many ways.

I sat patiently and listened for the Lord to share the insight to the current events surrounding us as a whole Nation & Worldwide community. Sweetly, the Lord reminded me of the declaration made prior to 2020 arriving. I, distinctly heard him say, "This is your Harvest year – double is your portion. Communicate intentionally, and proactively prepare for what you expect to harvest." I was awestruck at the concise and clear instructions received that I planted the words very deeply in my heart. As David said: *Thy word have I hid in my heart, that I might not sin against thee.* Psalm 119:11 (KJV)

As I was overjoyed, hearing the positive & motivating declarations straight from Heaven, within days, several trials & turn of events occurred back-to-back. Immediately, testing and trying of my faith came to prevent the magnificent word from rooting deep in my soul. My trials consisted of untruthful and unsubstantiated statements from an insurance company handling a pending injury claim, which could jeopardize my job, benefits, and reputation. My integrity and livelihood were hanging in the balance. My spiritual place of worship was also in tribulation with some members feeling the pressure of life & fearful from information around the coronavirus, that they began choosing secular means for self-gratification. The term "walking by faith" was mocked as a joke or Neanderthal-style concept versus an encouraging word. Even some walked away physically, as well as emotionally, due to fear and anger in their hearts from losing their jobs and secure income.

Personally, I wanted to transfer to a position closer to my home, but was unable to post due to the current status of leave of absence due to an injury ... all these experiences in a short period of time, were taking a toll on me mentally, physically and spiritually.

So, as I teach others that when our hearts are overwhelmed and before we begin to follow the steps of insecurity and rationality, always rely on the Holy Scriptures to comfort and guide us on life's pathway ... Therefore, as I turned to the Bible (Basic Instructions Before Leaving Earth), the words lifted off the pages of the Bible and penetrated my heart at the precise areas needed as follows:

There was a famine in the land besides the first famine that was in the days of Abraham. 12 Then, Isaac sowed in that land and reaped in the same year hundredfold; And the Lord blessed him. 13 And the man waxed great, and went forward, and grew until he became very great: (Genesis 26:1,12,13 KJV)

I allowed these words not only to sink deeply in my heart, but I proliferated these words into action. The clear and concise instructions and activity began to take shape in my life. As people were hunkering down for self-survival mode, my heart was moved to reach out to the community even the more. We opened the church with online services along with Sunday live services held under tents & the portico. Amazing events began to spark, where people congregated also in the yards, driveways, and porches for fellowship to listen to the Word of God. Without requesting, the community voluntarily gave love donations just to say thank you for walking by faith during these pandemic times.

Moreover, the door was flung wide open not just to receive a transfer, but I was promoted to a higher position, given a window view office closer to my home along with a significant pay increase. A new company was assigned to my case with an apology for my treatment. Now, all this happened within two weeks of the entire state closing. I just don't consider this a blessing, but a miracle, during a time when businesses were laying off due to the slow economy.

The walk of faith and obedience stride, perfectly, together hand-in-hand. In my heart I heard a small voice say, "Don't walk by fear from your past but faith. This is not a repeat of 2008, for you were under an economic recession and famine. I want you to go forth and demonstrate your faith in My Words by paying off your car loan & credit card debt."

Logically, a person should save during famine or economic decline, but I was also pressed to give more in outreach like food, clothes, and toilet paper/paper towels to share in the burdens of others so they could see Hope & Faith in God & Humanity.

By walking by faith and trusting in the Lord, my household finances, health and well-being improved significantly. In addition to gaining new territory through my employment, I gained relationships within the community. I have received so many blessings of support from family and friends -- each time for giving & my obedience.

Success also overflowed into my hobbies as a Mary Kay consultant, Glow Time with Dr. J podcast, along with a request for an exclusive interview for Johnson Counseling Enrichment Center's upcoming launch.

Remembering all those who have survived and conquered the coronavirus, I commend you and implore you to plant seeds today, so you will reap a powerful, overflowing, and prosperous harvest tomorrow. *Those who sow with tears will reap in joy.* (Psalm 126:5)

Humbly submitted,

April L. Johnson, PhD, Christian Counseling
Drapriljohnson@protonmail.com
Plant City, FL 33563

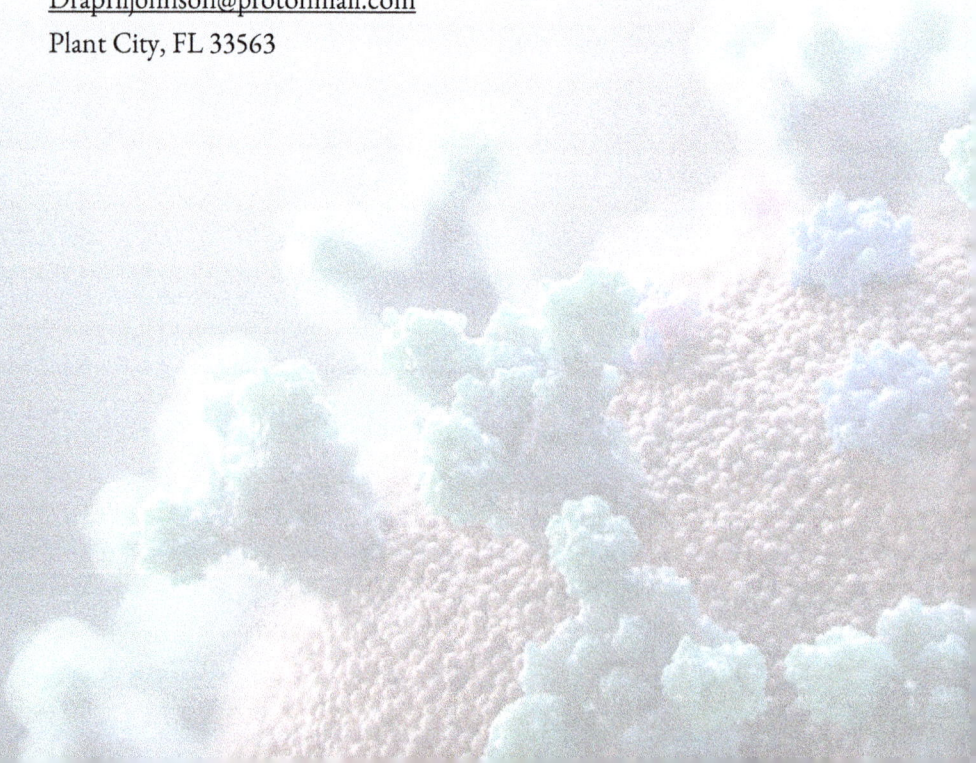

This concludes *Confinement Chronicles, Volume IV* – "My Mental Health During This Pandemic."

As we now end Volume IV, we encourage you to order Volumes I, II & III, and follow CONFINEMENT CHRONICLES by Angie BEE Productions on Facebook. As this series grows, we pray that you share them with others and learn from them, as well.

There were three times when I tried to end my life. Mental illness had me in its grasp, and I felt as though I was all alone. Fortunately for me, in the State of Florida, people like me become hospitalized, and there, I learned coping skills which helped me to survive. If you or someone you know is feeling lost, don't wait to "snap out of it." Seek medical attention, seek counseling, seek help from the scriptures, and cry out to the Lord. It helped me, and we want it to help you, too.

Be safe and BEE Blessed
Sincerely,

Evangelist Angie BEE

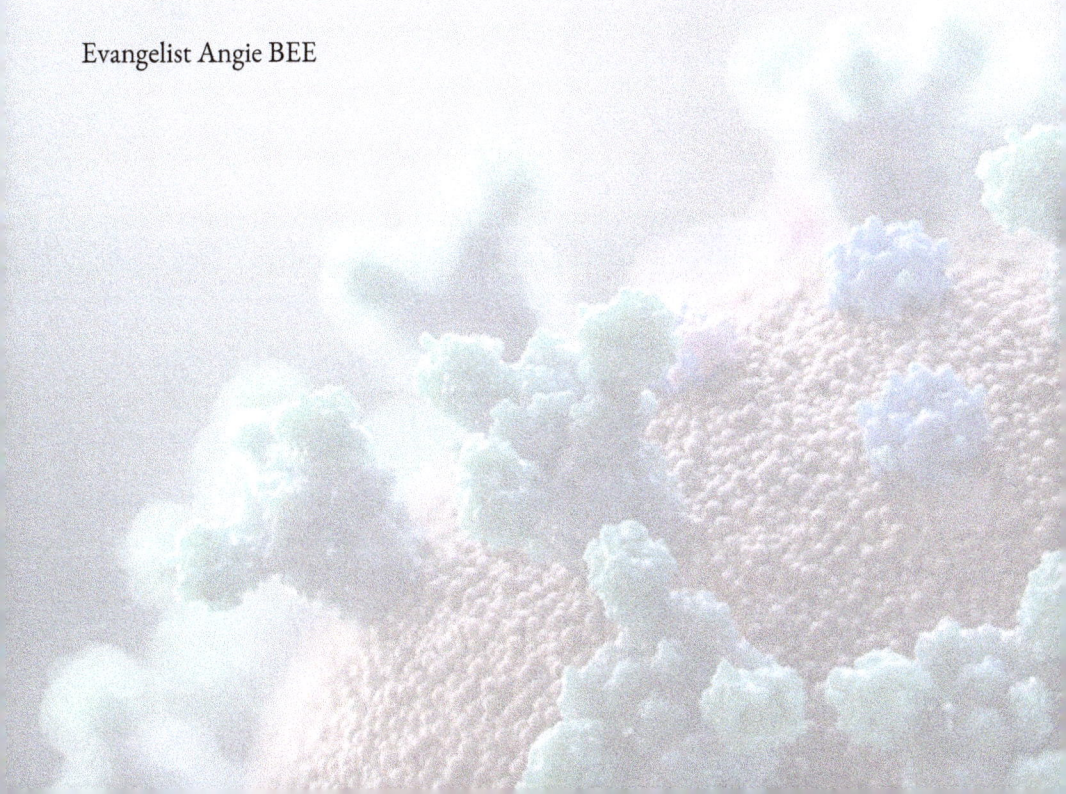

VOLUME V

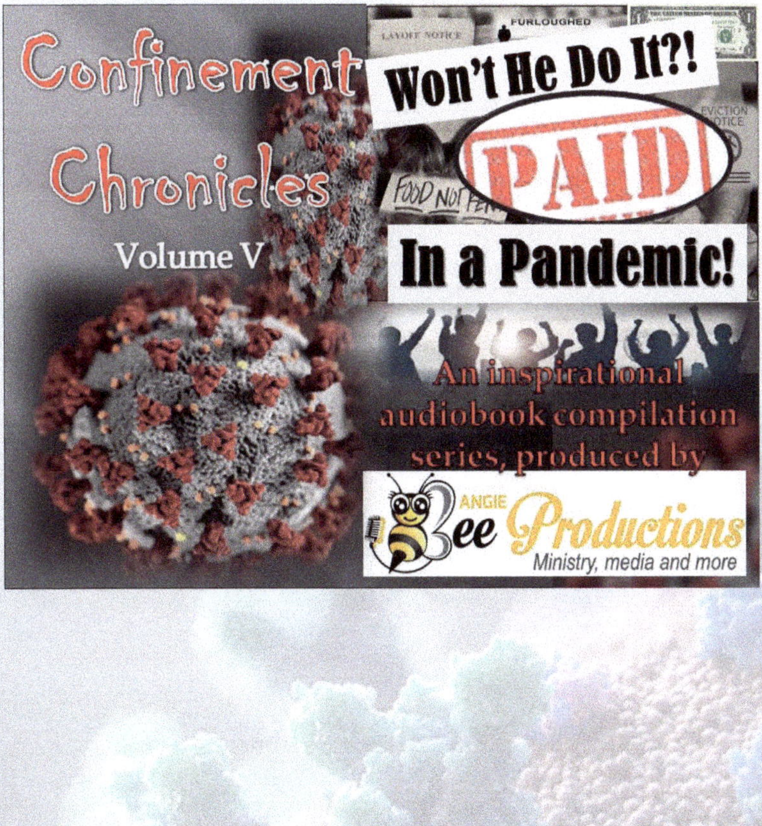
Confinement Chronicles
Volume V
Won't He Do It?!
PAID
In a Pandemic!
An inspirational audiobook compilation series, produced by
ANGIE Bee Productions
Ministry, media and more

I Found My Purpose and Now I am Pushing Forward

Tamara MackRoy

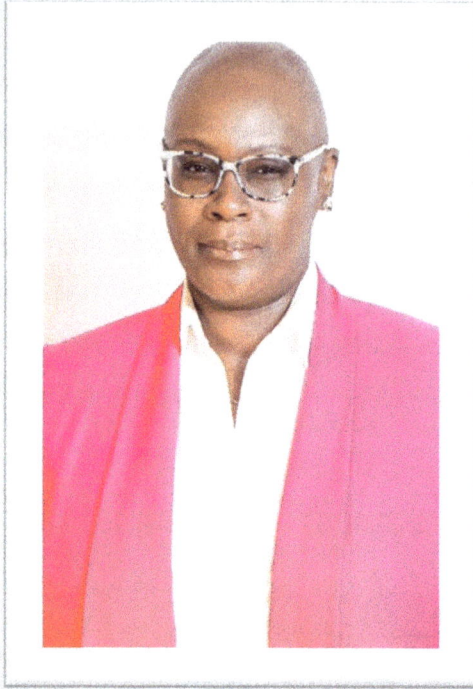

Hi, Tamara here from Management & Consultative Favor (MaCFavor) Here to speak to you about finding your purpose and pushing forward in it during this pandemic. I have always been a Corp America employee, and in this pandemic, I decided to quit my job as a Program Manager. I was making great money, had excellent employees, and was burning myself out.

I realized the peace of mind in pursuing what God placed in me was greater than chasing a FAT paycheck. When God has a calling on your life, He will repeatedly tap you on your shoulder about it. He will close doors that you know you are

QUALIFIED to walk into. You will learn to humble yourself and become attuned to His word.

It is NOT easy. At this present moment, I do not know where my rent, car note, light, etc. bill money is coming from. BUT the truth is, as a child of God, you will NOT lack in your obedience. I am constantly excited about the means that God is making in my life. It's called having faith. You see, God gave me a gift. I have been working my business as a part-time gig since 2016. As my book-of-business started to grow, in 2018, God spoke to me and told me to give the business an official name and formalize the business structure. So, I incorporated the business through a website and printed some business cards. Still chasing after a "fat check", I neglected MaCFavor until May of 2019, when I was laid off.

Me being me, I took time to listen to God, grew the business a little, and then returned to Corp America. God being God tapped on my shoulder again and questioned me on my happiness, peace of mind, and the Will He has for my life. That is when I quit my j-o-b July of 2020. Here it is September, and I am still lacking nothing. My business is growing, and my peace of mind is better than it has been in years. Working with Human Services Providers throughout the nation to help them build healthier business operations is what I thrive off of. It is something I have been doing since the late 90s (not to date myself).

I tell you all of this to say, please KNOW that in this era of a pandemic, God is still slaying. His Word has never gone void. You can make it. If you are doing His will ...

WE ARE MORE THAN CONQUERERS!

Theresa Jordan

Founder and Publisher of *Triumphant Magazine*

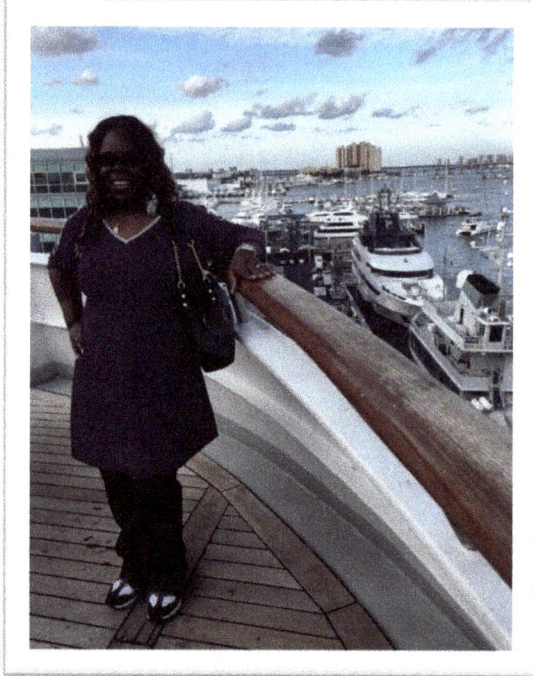

Triumphant Magazine is a stronger presence nationally, and God has enabled me and my publishing associates to thrive and flourish in this season. I am so grateful because during these unprecedented times, we are blessed to have a stronger digital media platform and stronger social media presence. It is amazing because most of our subscribers prefer the online version of *Triumphant*. Now, we are still fortunate to have readers prefer having the hard copies, but both requests are greatly appreciated. Our online presence has intensified, and that is a true blessing indeed. The Lord is expanding the borders of *Triumphant Magazine*, and He is enlarging her territory.

God has blessed me in gigantic ways because I have been blessed to work with *Confinement Chronicles*, and I now have seven audiobooks through *Confinement Chronicles* with Angie BEE Productions. The Audiobooks are phenomenal, and they have been inspired by God. Please feel free to contact us directly to get yours; they are only fifteen dollars each.

Triumphant Magazine is an extraordinary magazine for extraordinary people, and we are willing to share triumphant moments with the world.

Triumphant Magazine is scheduled to launch its store through e-commerce, so it is coming soon. God has blessed me tremendously during this season, and He has allowed me to not lack any good thing. Let me share some details with you:

1. I have had several opportunities to go back to school through Facebook and several other platforms.
2. I have been blessed to attend several conferences that would have charged an enormous amount of money had this pandemic not occurred in 2020.
3. I have attended several free virtual conferences and workshops all over the world and during the month of October, *Triumphant Magazine* will celebrate our three-year anniversary as a publication! In other words, instead of everything requiring a hotel, money, building, or hotels; businesses closing and major corporations handing out layoff notices, God proved that He is able to make a way out of no way! God continues to make provisions for my husband and me, our children, family, and friends. If I had to calculate how much I would have been charged without this pandemic existing in 2020, it would have been over twenty thousand ($20,000). But God has the tendency of making the impossible possible in my life every day. Matthew 19:26 tells me, *But Jesus beheld them, and said unto them, with men this is impossible; but with God all things are possible.*
4. Since the pandemic, *Triumphant Magazine* has launched our first Podcast entitled: "Triumphant Moments." We are blessed to come on

twice (Tuesdays & Thursdays), and we can be found on anchor.fm/Theresa-jordan4. We can also be found on Spotify, Radio/Public podcast, and several other podcast and radio platforms.

5. We recently launched our YouTube page, and we can be found on https://youtube.com/channel/UCeo3p90XpJ-zAHRH76fEE2Q

6. All I can say is "To God Be the Glory, Honor, and Praise." *Triumphant Magazine* reminds me of the song called, "Jacob's Ladder," because every round the good Lord continues to go higher and higher in the name of Jesus. *Triumphant Magazine* is blessed to experience this firsthand by the grace of the Great Almighty, and He is taking her higher and higher every year.

I have been blessed to become a coach, so now I am Coach Theresa Jordan through Ultimate Coaching Exchange. God is allowing my cup to run repeatedly; we are in the process launching two new websites for *Triumphant Magazine*, which is Triumphantmagazine.com and Jordan Destinations & Event Planning, which is Jordandestinations.com. God has been an excellent provider, and he has blessed my husband, Daniel, to be an excellent provider.

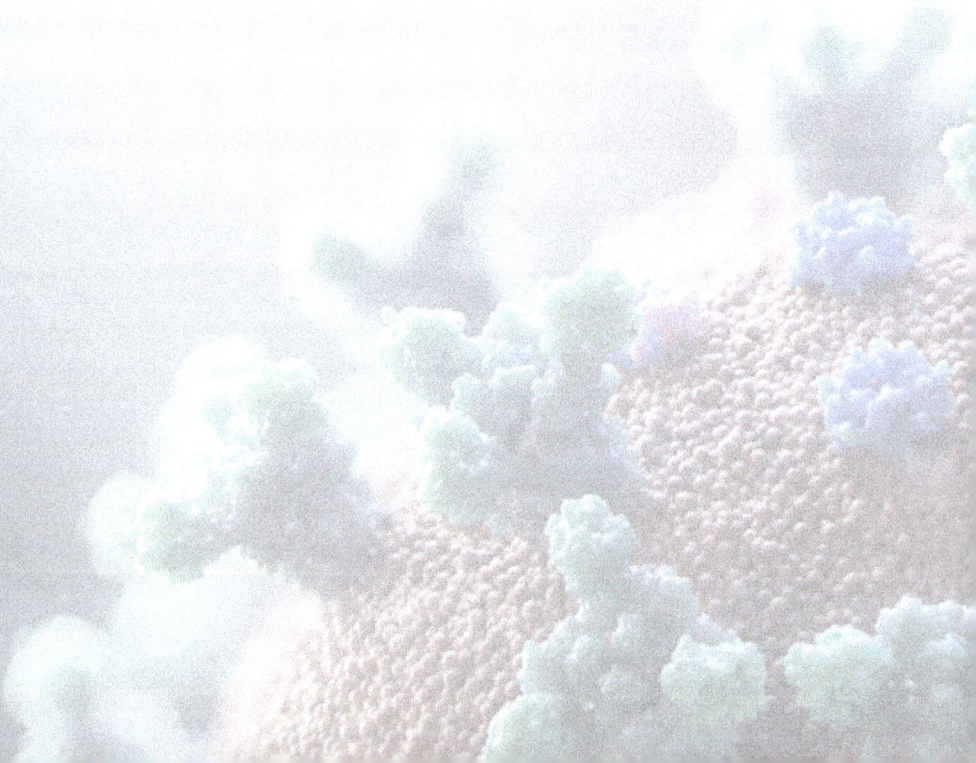

THEY DOO-ED!

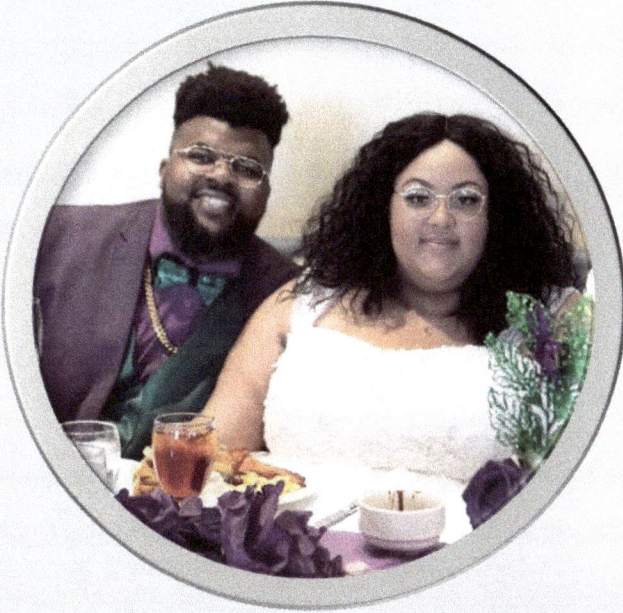

The following story was written by Angie BEE and is dedicated to Ric &
Rainbow. Their love story, wedding and subsequent happy marriage, in spite of
the pandemic, has been an encouragement for all that know them.

On February 29th, I was honored to officiate the wedding of my youngest daughter "Rainbow", to her fiancé "Ric." As with most weddings, we are all now anxiously awaiting the official portraits to arrive from the wedding photographer. I just know that these images will be spectacular, as Rainbow's beloved Aunt served as official photographer. Oh, how her Auntie expressed true love for Rainbow and Ric on that day, and we can't wait to see that love reflected in the images that she captured!

The weekend was filled with love as friends and family arrived via buses, planes, changed vacation plans, drove, and were driven in to witness this act of love between Ric and Rainbow. Sacrifices were made, hearts were mended, and the ocean breeze tried to blow us away (LOL!) My prayer partners were on hand to minister to me; my phone was ringing with offers of prayers and love; and as I witnessed my youngest child prepare to be given away to this man, *I managed not to shed one tear during the service.* PRAISE GOD!

Then, COVID-19 hit the world. The death toll grew, the world began to change and even the churches began to close their doors. People are instructed not to gather together in groups, and my eldest daughter gave God praise that her sister's wedding took place BEFORE the virus hit!

Have you felt loved lately? Have you shown love toward anyone lately?

Our family wedding was a loving occasion, and the way our family is now supporting one another during this Coronavirus is a true act of love.

God loved us, and He loves us. Even through this pandemic, there are acts of love all around us. The pollen count is high: this means that God is preparing for new plants, flowers, and trees to grow. Weddings are still taking place, and women are still getting pregnant (I'm sure there will be a few babies named after Coronavirus or the Pandemic after this is all over). This means that new families are growing and still being blessed by God. How do you "celebrate" Easter, with the churches closing? Bless someone in your family! Cook and deliver a meal to a senior citizen. Write a lesson plan and email it to that single mother's child. Show someone else that the Love of Jesus is alive IN YOU, and make your act of love that *memorable* act they will remember for a lifetime!

**Now, let me share with you the testimony from the newlyweds,
"Ric and Rainbow"**

On a cold-windy-sunny Saturday, February 29, 2020, I married my best friend, on the beach on Amelia Island, Florida. We were surrounded by friends and family, and the day could not have been more perfect for us! Then, COVID-19 hit, and the world shut down a week later. I think about the people that lost their jobs, homes, relatives, spouses, and their lives; but we are still together.

We still have a roof over our head, and our car is still on the road. We still cook and dine out. We still visit with relatives, and we are still in love. We even have two new additions to our family: July and Yuri, our turtles ... LOL. To say that this first year of "wedded bliss" has been challenging would be an understatement, but we are still here! We are still standing tall, and we want this story to be an inspiration to another!

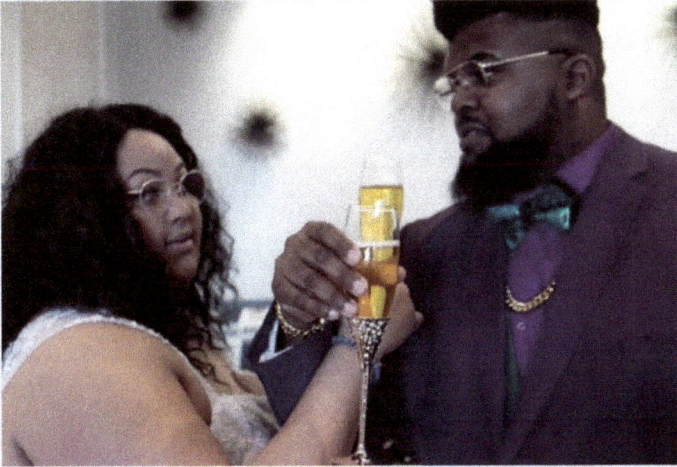

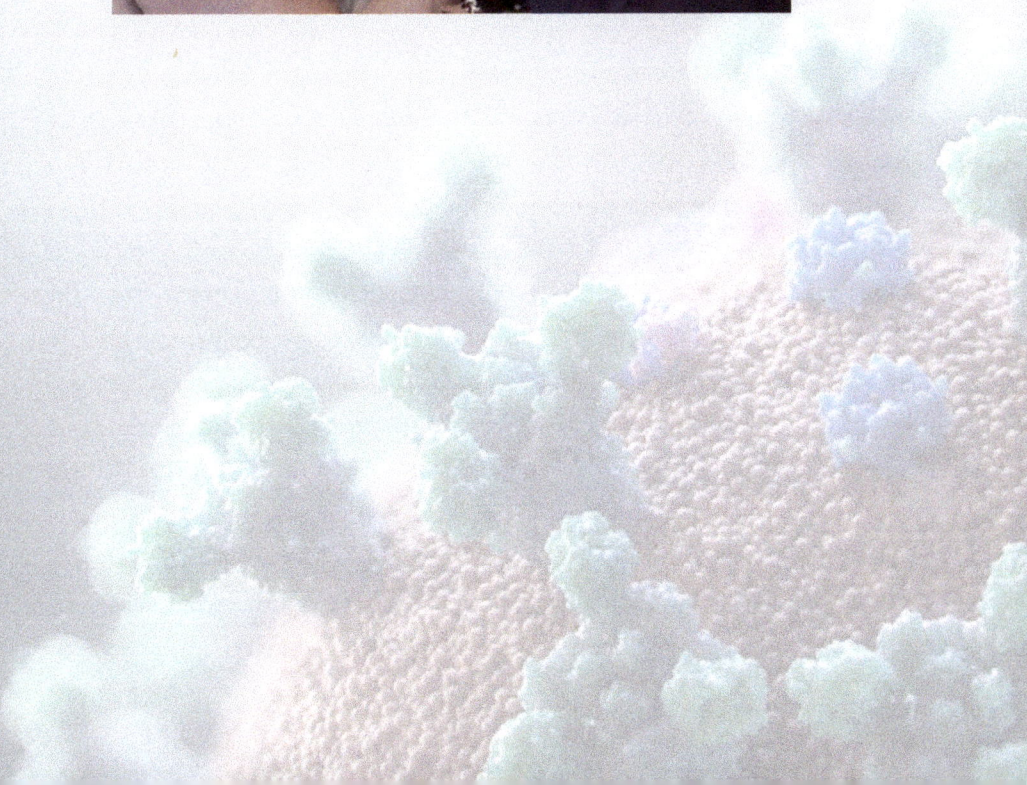

BOUNTIFUL BLESSINGS IN A PERILOUS PANDEMIC

An Anonymous Church Member

In a time when lives are being threatened and lost by a virus obtained from everyday activity, jobs eliminated, and mental health shaken, my memories of 2020 will be of the generosity shown by unusual sources. Who would have thought that *toilet paper* would be a hoarder's dream -- a commodity like a cigarette in prison?

Instead of curling up in despair as school buildings closed (forcing a rise in unemployment), I thanked God for the internet. For years, I've heard people talk about "free money", and I would unsuccessfully seek these 'unicorns of cash' out, only to fall behind the eight ball in researching their legitimacy. My attention would revert back to work, motherhood, and adult responsibilities that fell in the path of potential posterity. Now, the world is my virtual oyster, and time is abundant under an Executive Order to stay put. Stimulus Deposits, Pandemic Unemployment Assistance, Paycheck Protection Plans -- all ripe for the picking, and I stood ready to seek out and pluck them off the internet like a gardener pulls the top of a carrot.

The first unexpected blessing was an unprecedented gratuity from the Government for all tax filers: a minimum of $1200.00 per household. Prior to hearing this, one of my parents-in-the-struggle (a tax professional) inquired whether I had filed my yearly taxes. Paralyzed in depression, I had not: believing my income -- for the first time in my adult life -- was insufficient for anything but surviving and rather than accrue *another* unavoidable bill, I had decided to ignore a lingering problem to an aggressive "Uncle." Two weeks after she finally convinced me that I wouldn't owe and that there were new deductions to ensure that, The Government announced these automatic deposits called "Stimulu$"

that would magically deposit into the bank accounts that the IRS accessed yearly. My small family was blessed with $1600.00 that I clung to like a pacifier.

Bountiful Blessings: Never Thought I'd See the Day!

Being a single parent, my external moneymaker was placed on hold when my daughter's education became an in-house assignment. Hello, M.A.R.V.I.N. (Michigan Automated Response Voice Interactive Network for Unemployment recipients); thought we were "broke" up long ago, never to rekindle, yet here we are: on a bi-weekly phone "date." Enter the PUA: a Pandemic Unemployment Assistance fund that allotted an additional certified $600.00 a week on top of the weekly unemployment amount. In addition, many of the unemployment-eligible restrictions were softened, and those of us who didn't know how they'd make it could now see the forest through the trees -- at least for a few months. Shortly after that fund was exhausted, FEMA stepped in with a $300.00 weekly stipend for a moment to help out those who were still struggling.

Next: PPP Grants from the Small Business Administration. As my personal blessings continued to flow, I began thinking of the business owners in my life that were also struggling and wondered if there was anything out there for them. Kind of as an, "I wonder if...", I applied for a Paycheck Protection Plan grant that I'd read a little about that would help cover employees' wages and utilities: business expenses for my favorite nonprofit -- my church. Since the doors closed and virtual services became a necessity -- not an option, they were suffering financially since our older congregation was unfamiliar and uncomfortable with electronic donating and passing the basket was temporarily not an option.

Having been sent for a grant-writing class by my Pastor the year before (God was *preparing* me), I re-read the parameters and requirements, gathered the necessary paperwork, and quietly applied. Juuussstt as I started wondering, "Hey, whatever happened to that application," my phone started ringing from Deacons, Trustees, and my Pastor asking if I knew where the $10,000.00 tax-free deposit into the church's checking account came from. You see: I didn't tell anyone, so as to not get hopes high, and since I had dabbled with grant applications after the class, I had the necessary information without asking anyone. My church was approved and "granted" ten thousand dollars that did not require repayment and was an initial amount subtracted from a $65,000.00 loan at a 2.3% interest rate that has <u>already</u> been forgiven! Just like that: wages, utilities, food bags, clothes, and much-needed renovations available for God's House from less than an hour of commitment of time.

Bountiful Blessings Expanded to a Community

Right after I pressed "Submit" on the church's application, an essential-worker friend shared that their work vehicle was in need of repair. I'm always leery of passing information before I've seen the fruits; however, THIS time, I told her and a few additional small businesses to apply and suggested, "The worse that can happen is you're denied, and then you're still scrambling; the best that can happen is you're approved and able to stay afloat." Each received a deposit used for business equipment, employee wages, and even the essential worker who was able to get vehicle repairs! Did I mention my entrepreneurial effort (that, like everything else I'd put on the backburner) also received a slice of the stay-afloat pie?

Bountiful Blessings for the Little (Wo)man

My County takes care of its residents and businesses. As part of the C.A.R.E.S. Act (the Coronavirus Aid Relief and Economic Security Act), the County I live in began to make grants available for household bills; brick and mortar business expenses; and even bills for businesses that one wouldn't think would, but does (such as entertainment), sustains our community. From this pot, my socially-aware small business was granted $2500.00 which I've used to revamp and update my business plan and product design. After an extensive application process, a grant became available for utility, mortgage and rent assistance -- providing a one-time payment of at least three months' worth of essential bill payments. Consequently, my lights and gas are well taken care of.

Bountiful Blessings: Protecting the Roof Over Our Head

As an extension of the household bill-grant and because I have a student in my home, I was contacted by an agency about our internet service. I was offered a year of free internet (to ensure my virtual learner would continue to excel) and informed that the mobile phone company offering this spectacular blessing would provide a reduced rate after the year promotion expires if we were to accept it. IF we were to accept it?! Our city is held hostage by one large cable company for internet services and their prices are reflective of the lack of options. I accepted this gracious offer (of course) and was then told that under this program, I'd receive a desktop printer and a laptop: for free, to keep! When an HP Color Printer showed up on my porch along with compatible ink cartridges and a ream of paper, I was beside myself!

Bountiful Blessings of Technology

Since becoming unemployed, I entered a twice-daily counseling session with a well-known, national charity that serves communities in several ways: warm meals, canned goods, cleaning supplies, trainings, and even a warm shower if needed. Through this Partner of Hope, I learned some financial training, explored some talents I had subdued for potential employment opportunities, and even learned to garden! During this pandemic, in-office contact was unavailable, so I emailed my counselor to ask if we could possibly have an outdoor meeting and, thankfully, that was allowed. In this casual and much-needed session, I casually mentioned that I'd recently lost two main teeth and that my speech and self-esteem were being affected. I also noted that I'd had the same glasses for about five-plus years and that I wondered if my prescription was altering due to the additional screen time both my daughter and I were doing. Not by coincidence, only by grace: this year's newest available assistance grant was for medical necessities up to $2000.00 which was more than enough for dental work and new glasses for both of us!!

Unforeseen Blessings that I could sink my teeth into (like my puns? ☺)

W hile many look forward to 2021 bringing change, hope, and medical miracles, I've continuously praised God in this moment for the lemonade He's provided from the lemons I've been given.

This concludes *Confinement Chronicles, Volume V – PAID in a Pandemic*.
As we now end Volume V, we encourage you to order Volume I, II, III, IV, VI, VII, VIII and IX and follow *Confinement Chronicles* by Angie BEE Productions on Facebook. As this series grows, we pray that you share them with others, and learn from them, as well. During our 2021 tour, come out to meet and network with us and let us know if this series was helpful to you.

Enjoy and BEE Blessed
Sincerely,

Evangelist Angie BEE

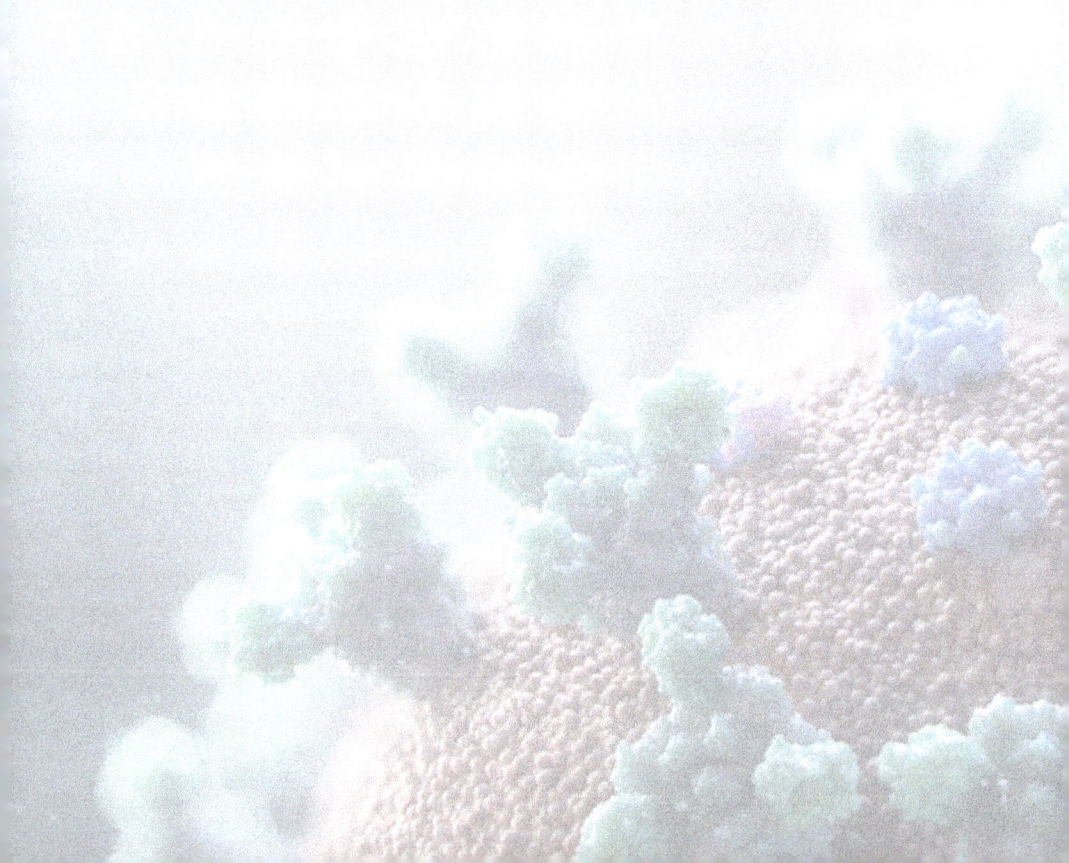

VOLUME VI

Confinement Chronicles

Volume VI

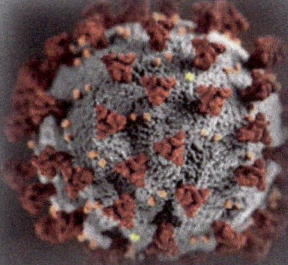

When the Doors of the Church Closed

An inspirational audiobook compilation series, produced by

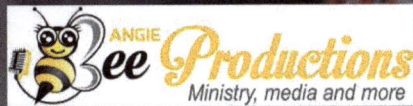

ANGIE Bee Productions

Ministry, media and more

A s the year 2020 approached, several ministry leaders made plans for "New Vision – Clear Vision & Clean Vision" events. There were conferences and workshops planned, revivals, and ribbon-cutting ceremonies, too. There were so many opportunities to invite "guests" to attend their service and save their souls once they crossed the threshold. I was invited to speak at several of these events, and then the pandemic hit.

In accordance with CDC guidelines that no more than ten people could gather together in a public place, churches all across the country had to cease holding services in their buildings. Some church leaders violated the orders, and they were seen on TV being arrested. Other church leaders left their church members to "fend for themselves" as they were not equipped to reach them if they weren't in the pulpit. A lot of church leaders began having "church" on social media – which forced many senior citizens to Facebook pages for the first time in their lives. It was then that the Lord placed upon my heart to produce a volume of this series entitled, "When the Doors of the Church Closed."

We felt that this volume would need to come from our church leaders. We wanted to hear what THEY had to say to reach their flock when the CDC forced their churches to close. We reached out to pastors, reverends, bishops and evangelists via social media. We emailed them; we "tagged" them, and we called them on the phone. We even offered to add their contribution without charging them the $25 submission fee! Some of them promised to write something; others never responded. Some needed to "think about it" and "pray over it" while others never even responded. In some cases, their "gate-keepers" never delivered the message to the church leaders, stating they were "busy" or "meditating" or "they never stopped having service, so the topic would be irrelevant."

And we also thank God continually because, when you received the word of God, which you heard from us, you accepted it not as a human word, but as it actually is, the word of God, which is indeed at work in you who believe.
1 Thessalonians 2:13

I have said these things to you, that in me you may have peace. In the world you will have tribulation. But take heart; I have overcome the world.
John 16:33

Now, don't get me wrong – I am not saying that you should not go to your Spiritual Leader in a time of crisis or when you need encouragement, but don't solely rely on them! They are people, too, and they are going through some of the same things that YOU are going through. During this pandemic, I know of pastors that lost their vision, lost their pulpit, lost their jobs, lost relatives and lost their lives. Don't sit and wait to hear from them – you need to reach out and encourage them, too!

But David strengthened himself in the LORD his God. – I Samuel 30:6

So, that is what we did! We encouraged the leaders of the church, and we prayed for them. As the result of our obedience, the Lord opened our hearts and minds to receive a word from HIM! Scriptures began to leap forth in my mind and on the page. People wrote encouraging stories filled with love from the Holy Spirit. I can't WAIT for you to hear what they wrote!

We have arrived at Volume VI and, although it may have been delivered to listeners a bit out of order (Volume VII debuted on September 1, 2020), these words that you are about to experience are WELL WORTH THE WAIT!

And now, for our first contribution...

WE SHOULD BE MAKING "CHURCH" INTO A CLASSROOM

Church was boring. Church was loud up in the front (the sanctuary). I resented being the eldest kid in the church, and if the younger kids got in trouble, everyone looked to me as if to say, "Where were YOU when this happened?" When the church doors closed because of COVID-19, I wasn't like "YOO HOO" because it was expected – everything was closed because of the virus, but I certainly was not disappointed because I didn't have to go.

When the doors of the church reopen, I would like to see more kids my age to help keep my time occupied. It would be cool to have more teens present. I go to church to spend more time with kids my age, but I know that really defeats the purpose because I wouldn't be in the sanctuary; I would be interacting with other kids. NOTHING IN THE SANCTUARY IS APPEALING TO ME! Not the choir, not the usher board, not the preaching.

If church was like English Language Arts (ELA), I would like it because of the interaction. In ELA we work in groups; we are called up to the board to answer questions and reflect on what was read. If church had more reading, getting your questions answered, and less structure, we would be making "church" into a classroom, and I might look forward to attending.

- Words from a teenager that chose to remain anonymous

CHURCH LEADERS!

Are you make plans to re-open the doors of your church? PLEASE make plans for your children and teens. Some of them are already attending under duress, and the lack of age-appropriate spiritual training and leadership is disappointing! Church is not a babysitting service, nor is it a place where you let your children run wild while you "serve." Church is a place that can give your children even more than you can give them IF the church is equipped to offer that "more." Church is what you contribute to it, not just for your family, but for your community, and to give glory.

It has been said that, "It takes a village to raise a child." Well, our neighbors aren't the village that they once were. Our "village" is the church! As a child, I was baptized at Beth Eden Missionary Baptist Church in Detroit, Michigan, and I was raised at Hartford Memorial Baptist Church in Detroit. I graduated from St. Mary's of Redford Catholic High School in Detroit and immediately departed to attend Wilberforce University, a private, coed, liberal arts historically black university (HBCU) that was affiliated with the African Methodist Episcopal (AME). As my career launched, I aligned my memberships with non-denominational congregations where I learned to combine each of my religious lessons into a solid relationship with Christ.

Baptist, Catholic, AME, and non-denominational religious training all led me to a life of servitude and pure spiritual evangelism. I don't take light of it! I thank my mother for aligning me with a church that catered to raising and educating the young people in the church. Let us give our youth attendees the solid foundation of learning to fall-in-love with the Word of God to help them avoid some of the pitfalls of life and reach others with love.

Due to the pandemic, many churches now offer their services online, on their website. If your church does NOT have a website, I advise you to get one! Your website could be the only "church" that someone has access to, and the only way they can find a word from God. Facebook is great, but I know people who don't have Facebook accounts. They opened an account JUST to watch your services, but they would have preferred to watch from the church's website. Get a website; stream from it. Launch a mailing campaign to send encouraging letters to our senior citizens and those without internet access, and stop relying on people to get up and come to the church.

DO THE WORK OF AN EVANGELIST!

But you should keep a clear mind in every situation. Don't be afraid of suffering for the Lord. Work at telling others the Good News, and fully carry out the ministry God has given you. 2 Timothy 4:5 *New Living Translation (NLT)*

~ Evangelist Angie BEE
Amazon #1 Best-Selling Author
Founder of the evangelism troupe "The TOUR that Angie BEE Presents"
Narrator & Lead Producer – Angie BEE Productions

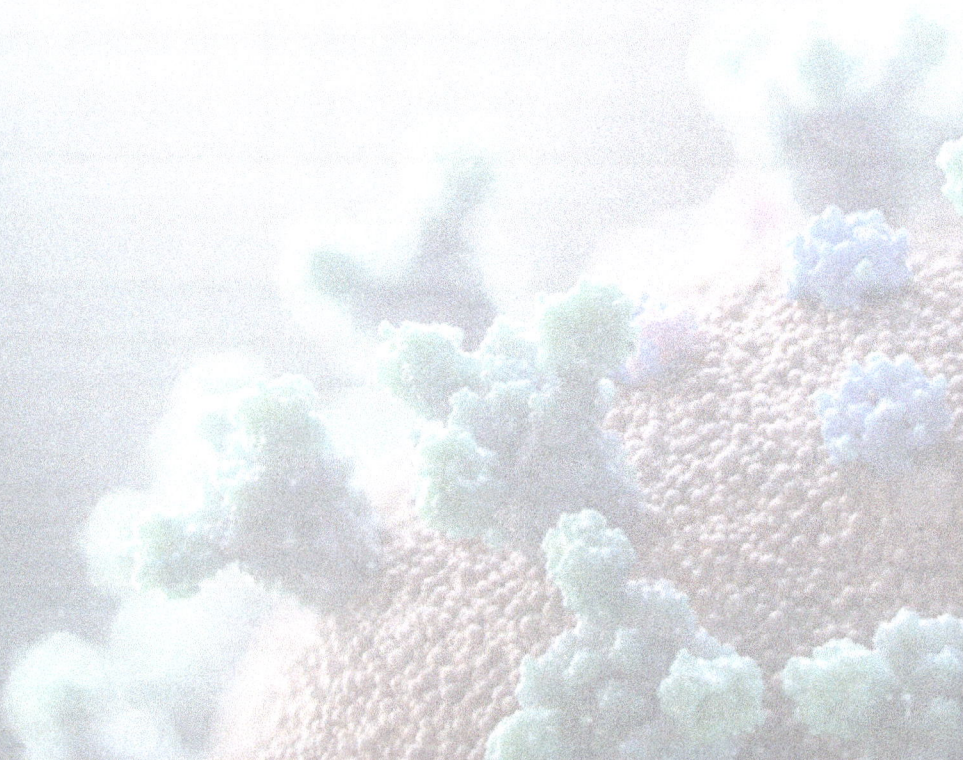

WHY IS THIS DOOR CLOSED?

Karen Chandler

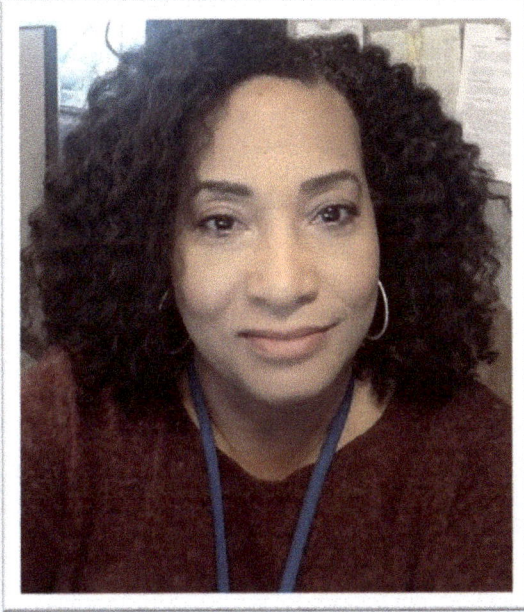

S ometimes, God will close a door because it's time to move forward. He knows you better than you know yourself. If needed, God will use circumstances to propel you forward. Trust God as you are going through!

We should be able to recognize when a season, job, or relationship is over. We should choose to depart from situations that we have outgrown. When we make the choice to move on, it doesn't have to be a disastrous or dramatic affair. We should simply choose to move forward with peace and clarity of mind.

God will close doors we are not supposed to go through. No man will be able to open them either. If it was meant for you, the door would be open. Here are some reasons that the door may be closed:

1. Defense from harm - Isaiah 54:17
   No weapon that is formed against you will prosper
2. Rerouting- He wants to make sure you go through the correct door. He is the ultimate GPS system.
3. God requires obedience from you. Did you follow His previous instructions?

The door God opens requires dependence on Him.

1. He insists that we put Him first. Matthew 6:33 (AMP)
   But first and most importantly seek (aim at, strive after) His kingdom and His righteousness [His way of doing and being right—the attitude and character of God], and all these things will be given to you also.
2. Open doors may require us to use our faith. Hebrews 11:6 (AMP)
   But without faith it is impossible to [walk with God and] please Him, for whoever comes [near] to God must [necessarily] believe that God exists and that He rewards those who [earnestly and diligently] seek Him. Open doors may require us to stretch our faith. He wants us to grow in faith and become more like Christ every day. The increase in faith will also assist us with things coming up in the future. If He is taking us to another level, it will require a higher level of faith in order to function.

We can confirm that the door is open for us:

1. Through His Word - Psalm 119:133 (AMP)
   Establish my footsteps in [the way of] Your word; Do not let any human weakness have power over me [causing me to be separated from You].
2. Godly counsel from others – Will simply be a validation that you are going in the correct direction.

God made us all to fulfill His perfect plan, will, and purpose. He will also direct us through every situation. We must be willing be to listen to his directions.

Prayer

Father, in the name of Jesus I come to you. I enter Your gates with thanksgiving and Your courts with praise. Lord, I thank You because Your Word says that the prayers of the righteous make tremendous power available. If I seek (aim at and strive after) the Kingdom of God and Your righteousness (Your way of doing and being right) then You will provide me with everything thing that I need.

The steps of a good man are ordered by the Lord, and You delight in his way. I'm becoming more like Christ every day. I will keep You first in everything that I do. Thank You Lord for being my GPS in this life here on earth.

I will follow Your voice only, a stranger's voice I will not follow. I have the mind of Christ. Your Word is hidden in my heart, so I will not sin against You. I am surrounded by godly men and women who provide me with godly counsel. I decree and declare You are opening doors that no man can shut and closing doors that no man can open. Thank You Lord for ordering my steps.

Thank You for protecting me from every evil work and for continuous protection against every seen and unseen danger. No weapon formed against me will prosper. Every tongue that rises up against me will be condemned. Your Word will not return void, it will accomplish every single thing that You sent it to do. You are the same yesterday, today and forever. I thank You Lord for never leaving me or forsaking me. You knew me before the foundation of the world. I will fulfill Your perfect plan, will, and purpose for my life. In Jesus' name I pray. Amen.

WHEN THE DOORS OF THE CHURCH WERE CLOSED

The Beautiful Evangelist Althea Chavers

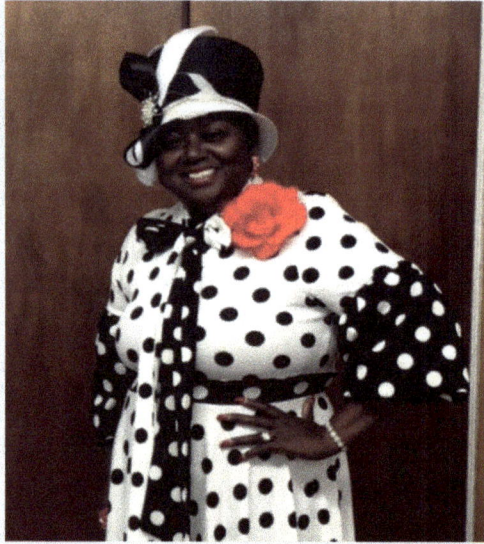

My name is Althea Ross Chavers, but I call myself The Beautiful Althea. I am the 1st Lady of the St. James Missionary Baptist Church in the City of Osteen, Florida, under the leadership of my husband, Rev. Larry D. Chavers Sr. We have been blessed to lead God's people for twenty-one years as of next month, November 2020.

When the doors of the church closed, I felt a little lost and discouraged, but after spending time with the Lord and talking with my daughter, we came up with a plan. We encouraged Pastor Chavers to do a conference call for our first service, especially since we were outside of the physical building. Several of our members are elderly, and they had no idea of how to connect with this new adjustment, but we attempted to make it work.

Our next effort was Facebook Live!!!

I was excited about using Facebook Live to stay connected with our members, and we were blessed to reach several people outside of our own flock.

We now have Facebook Live Sunday Service at 3:00 PM, and this takes place every Sunday. We have Facebook Live Bible Study on Thursdays at 7:00 PM, we call it "Thursday Night Live."

When the doors of the church closed, Christians had to think differently, and we had to become more creative with God's help and His guidance. Technology became our new best friend.

I am grateful to be under the leadership of a God-fearing man of God especially during these times. Pastor Chavers has given me the opportunity to share the Word of God to the people of God, and my husband and I and our children call ourselves TeamChavers.

We have been able to encourage God's people during these challenging times, and that is such an honor. We encourage the people of God by sending out weekly text messages to stay connected with each other. This encourages our members to send encouraging messages to each other.

We recognized the physical doors are closed, but we the people are the church, and just like Kirk Franklin says, "We Ain't Going Nowhere." We are God's servants, and we will continue to remain steadfast and unmovable, always abounding in the work of the Lord. We have had the opportunity to provide the elderly with fresh fruits, vegetables, and meat. The most rewarding part is seeing the smiles on our members' faces because it makes my heart smile.

In 1st Timothy 5, Paul describes the church as people dedicated to doing whatever it takes to reach out and help others.

I am honored to work with a man of God, my Pastor, my husband, outside of the four walls of the church to spread love and encouragement to God's people.

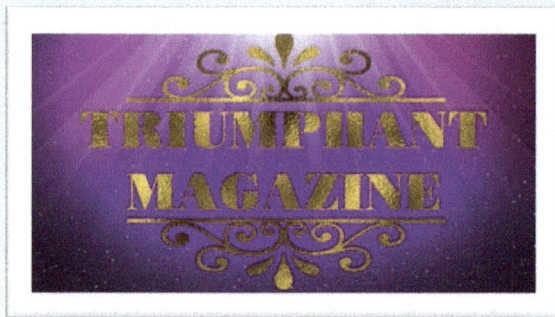

The following statement was originally written for Volume VII of our inspirational audiobook series *Confinement Chronicles – Out of the Mouths of Our Babes.* We invite you to relish in the words written by Theresa Jordan, Amazon #1 Best-Selling Author and publisher of *Triumphant Magazine.*

OUT OF THE MOUTHS OF BABES

I have watched several videos showing these pure conversations that were coming out of the mouths of our children. One video showed this adorable girl, and she was missing church so much she decided to have church on her own. This precious little baby repeatedly read Psalm 23 in its entirety,

1 The Lord is my shepherd; I shall not want.
2 He maketh me to lie down in green pastures: he leadeth me beside the still waters.
3 He restoreth my soul: he leadeth me in the paths of righteousness for his name's sake.
4 Yea, though I walk through the valley of the shadow of death, I will fear no evil: for thou art with me; thy rod and thy staff they comfort me.
5 Thou preparest a table before me in the presence of mine enemies: thou anointest my head with oil; my cup runneth over.
6 Surely goodness and mercy shall follow me all the days of my life: and I will dwell in the house of the Lord forever.

I know the baby's mother had been diligently teaching her little baby the ways of the Lord, and the mother had to be overjoyed videotaping this fascinating and powerful story to share with the world. If I had to guess the baby's age, it would be between 4 months and 8 months. The sincerity of witnessing this was breathtaking because this came forth out of the mouth of this astounding little girl. I was left flabbergasted again because this was coming forth out of the mouth of babes.

This is what I am talking about! When the doors of the church closed, these "babies" (according to Theresa Jordan) still had the Word of God within them, and are sharing their lessons globally.

How many of your sermons have reached outside of the four walls of the "church" building where they were delivered? I know this may sound harsh to some, but I pray these words are enlightening to others! Don't let the Word of God fall on "ears" that don't know how to "see" past the routine and "speak" that love to another. – Evangelist Angie BEE

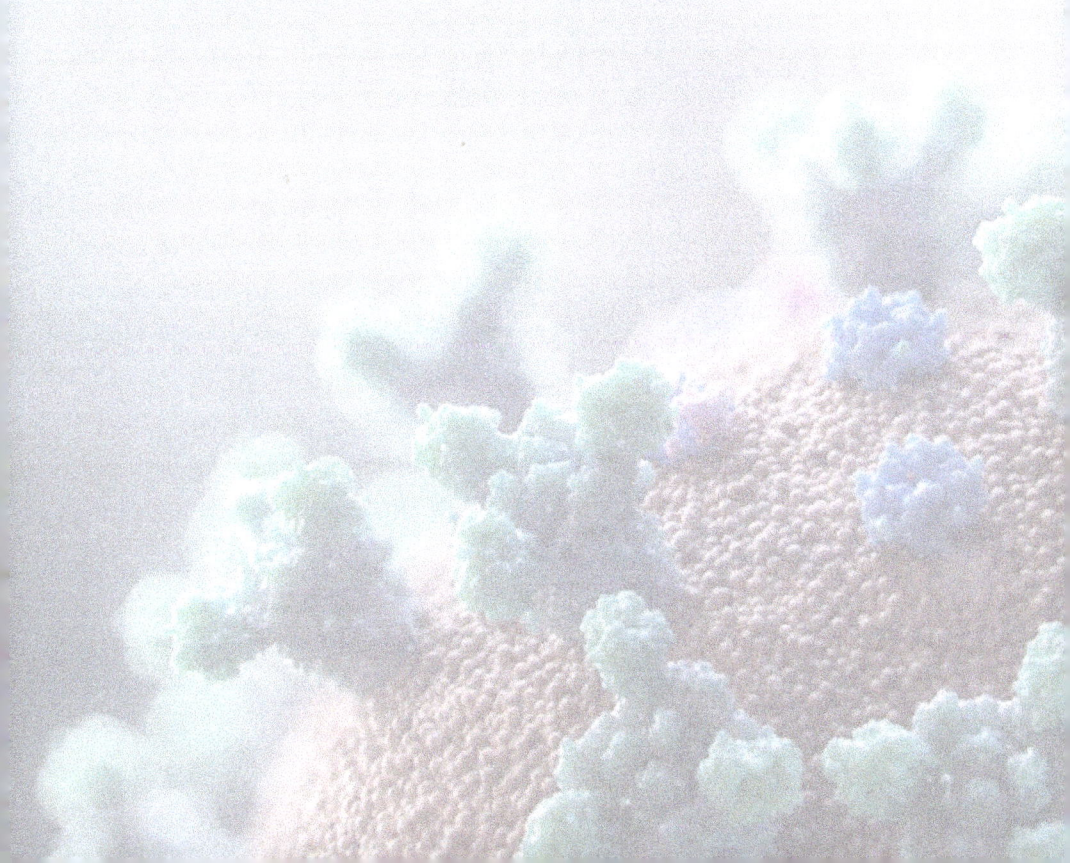

WHEN THE DOORS OF
THE CHURCH WERE CLOSED

Theresa Jordan

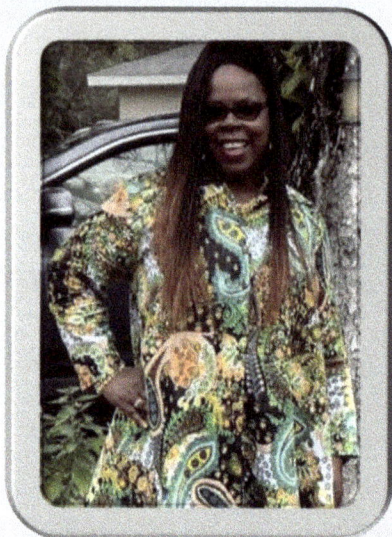

Our church doors closed the middle of March 2020, and the leaders at our church showed true leadership. The churches closing around the world reminded me of the Book of Revelation, and the profound stories I have heard throughout my life attending church. For instance, I remember hearing that there would come a time where the Saints of God would want to go to church, but they would not be able to attend church at all. I know that in theory we are considered the church, even though we are accustomed to going to the physical building. Bishop Paul Morton has a song called, "Bow Down and Worship Him." Within the song, it says, "This is holy ground, and we must worship Him." We know the Word tells us that **Faith** comes by hearing the Word of God (Romans 10:17), and I know we need to have a preacher because they are constantly watching and praying for our souls. God's word says, *Not forsaking the assembling of ourselves together, as the manner of some is but*

exhorting one another: and so much the more, as ye see the day approaching.
(Hebrews 10:25)

But if we walk in the light, as he is in the light, we have fellowship one with
another, and the blood of Jesus Christ his Son cleanseth us from all sin.
(1 John 1:7)

I must admit 2020 has been a new year for clear vision and putting things into
its proper perspective. Fortunately, God has assured us that through it all, we
can put our trust in Him. It has been declared in His Word, *And we know that*
all things work together for good to them that love God, to them who are the called
according to his purpose. (Romans 8:28)

I can honestly say that I have missed fellowshipping with my church St. James,
our Pastor and Evangelist, and the church family. We love each other
unconditionally, and we absolutely love serving and praising the Lord. These are
some of the things that would take place at our church:

First Sunday
Our deacon and mothers would do service together. The mothers would have
on the white dresses or two-piece suits. Our deacon would have on his black suit
with a white shirt and tie. Someone would say a powerful prayer, and a couple
of songs would be rendered, and a scripture would be read. My pastor or
Evangelist would deliver a dynamite word to the waiting congregation.

Second Sunday
The Distinguished Woman of God would lead the devotional service, and we
would sing a couple of songs, pray, and read a scripture.

Third Sunday

The mothers of the church would come back again and render songs and praises to the Lord. The mothers of the church would have on their elegant red dresses or two-piece suits, and some of them would have the audacity to wear their beautiful elegant red hats. The mothers at our church are always looking like they are jumping right out of the inside or off the cover of *Triumphant Magazine*. A couple of the mothers would do the prayer, and one of the mothers would read the scripture. We have one of our mothers that pulls out very meaningful songs from her personal archives each and every time, and here are some of the songs that she sings: "What is This", "Send Me", "I Will Go", "He Said", and "This Morning When I Rose." These songs I have mentioned are sung by various artists, and these songs are equivalent to having some homemade roast cooking in a slow cooker, rice, and beans that you are anticipating having for dinner after church service. The hymns and songs stick to you indefinitely, and trust me, God allows His precious Holy Spirit to bring everything back to our remembrance when you need it most. These songs I have are full of great substance, and they are worth reverting to, and it does not matter what season you are facing in life. Now please do not get me wrong, I love gospel music, and here are some of my favorite artists: Kirk Franklin, Brent Jones, Tasha Cobbs, J.J. Hairston, William Murphy, Jekalyn Carr, Mary Mary, and Yolanda Adams. I have several more, but this is just to name a few amazing singers to me.

When looking at the trajectory of everything that has taken place throughout this year, it gives everyone an opportunity to hear God's Word. It gives everyone a chance to hear from various churches around the world, and all of this is taking place because the church doors are closed. Churches have a chance to go beyond the physical building, and this enables the Word of God to reach the four corners of the earth. God promised in His Word, *And I, if I be lifted up from the earth, will draw all men unto Him.* (John 12:32) This is a pivoting time for Christians because it is bringing us closer to God, and it is bringing the ones who might have left the safety of the Lord back to Him. And the ones who might not have a relationship with our Lord. The church doors being closed allowed all of us to correct wrongs and ask the Lord for forgiveness. The church doors being closed provided a chance through these circumstances for us to get a right standard with

CONFINEMENT CHRONICLES | 119

God, and the ability to come back to our first love, which is Jesus Christ. God is performing a new thing in the season, and He is teaching us how to put Him first and how to put things back into their proper perspective when it comes to our churches, marriages, homes, families, businesses, neighbors, and schools.

It felt differently not going to church, but these adjustments were necessary. It forced leaders and many of us to start thinking quickly, and we started implementing things outside of the box. Our church started having services on Thursdays and Sundays on Facebook. Churches made changes quickly, and this displayed what true leaders are. There is a quote that I heard in the past and it states, "Good leaders come forth when things are challenging." In other words, it is easy to be a leader when things are going smoothly, but what makes a leader more illuminating is when they can maintain their leadership during unprecedented times just like the ones we are facing now. Leaders are relied on greatly to lead the way, and they have done an impeccable job with leaning on God's wisdom and understanding. We have adjusted and adapted well, and in closing, having the churches closed has provided advantageous ways of reaching people outside of the four walls. Because now we can attend several church services for Bible Study and church services. I know personally I am watching three-to-four different services on Sunday. This door of church being closed has impacted our lives tremendously because under normal circumstances this would not be possible. But God! He has sustained us for the entire of 2020, and may He be with us beyond.

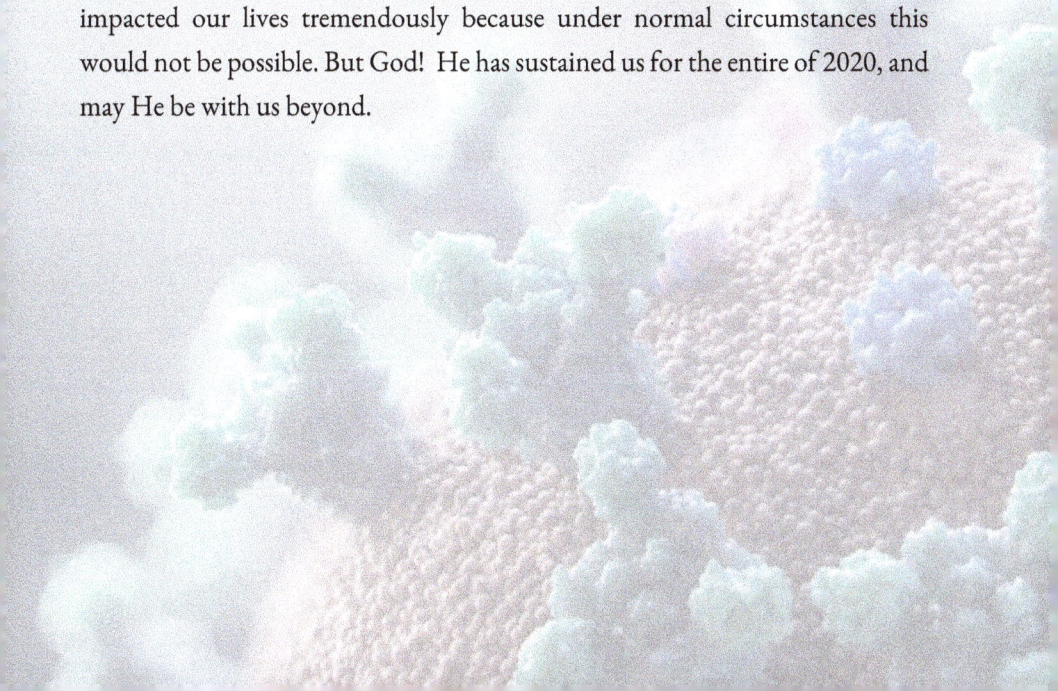

"IN OR OUT" – RIGHT OR WRONG?

Reverend Dawn Martin

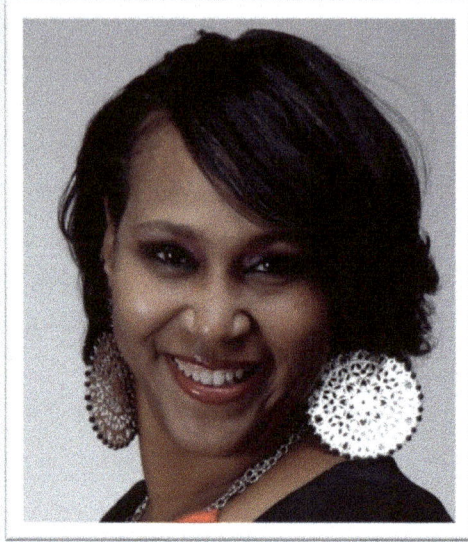

This is an unprecedented time, and with everybody so busy and trying to figure out what the "new busy" is for their lives during the pandemic, I thought it would be fitting to do it this way because this is where the world has gone: video meetings, Zoom meetings, and video chats are how we are conducting business during this pandemic. So, when asked to be a part of this wonderful book of minds, it took me a minute but I got there.

I am Dawn Martin from Dayton, Ohio, the Founder of Girls Empowered and Mentored to Success, as well as, the Risen Empowered Resource Center, and also the author of *Fill My Cup: Transitioning to Your Purpose*. So, when the question was asked about how did the pandemic affect church, I had to just take a breath. I can't tell you how many arguments and how many conversations I've been in the last seven months about this very topic.

For me, personally, I belong to what's called a semi-mega church; we have about fifteen hundred to two thousand members at our church, and so most of them, like any other urban church, are predominantly women which means there's a lot of elderly. There's a lot of women coming with comorbidity so they're already coming with their own health issues. We don't leave out the guys, there are some guys that are in the same boat that we're in, but when we're thinking about how, especially the black church, is affected by this pandemic, the black church is like the pillar of us as a culture. So ... What? We can't assemble? First of all, when you're thinking Biblically, that's against God, right? So, the biggest arguments and biggest clashes that I've had – some really good conversations with really some old-school saints have been right around that idea of how can you sit and say that you are Christian and you're not willing to assemble? You don't have faith! It depends on the level of faith you have. All of these things have been topics of discussion I've had over the last seven months when it comes to the response of the church to this pandemic.

My dad has been preaching for sixty to seventy years. He and I have had some really heated discussions because old-school is that the doors of the church never close. So, how dare you, Black Church, close the doors during this pandemic? We're not supposed to be about the world's business, we're supposed to be about God's business, and we're not supposed to operate ourselves based on the world's standards. We are in the world, not of the world (as my dad would say), so that just came up with so many conversations that it's like, "I understand Dad, but listen." The old school saints, the mindset is, "God is going to cover me." I can't say it's not true to a certain degree because my dad has a whole lot of things going on, and he is still assembling the way his church is allowing him to assemble. He does not attend my church, and he does not attend a church the size of my church, so that could be different. Their church is community; it has been able to get everybody in the parking lot of their church, so they have been doing a lot of parking-lot worshipping over the summer months. I think that's fantastic if you can figure out a way, to work it out that's best for your congregation – to keep your congregants as healthy and safe, as you could possibly do that, then by all means, meet in that parking lot and praise God out on that street. I am not arguing that; I have not said anything against any of that, but it's so interesting how I find myself defending my pastor's way to take care of me. Right?

So, in the beginning of the pandemic, you heard of all the churches that were still getting together, and the thousands of people who have lost their lives on top of thousands of people who have had to battle the illness and are still – post-illness – having symptoms left over that they are still dealing with -- all because the doors of the church didn't close. They were still telling their congregants to come to church in the middle and the height of this pandemic. It was just an epicenter for the disease to go all the way around. On top of that, everybody didn't wear masks then, so let's also keep that in place.

You have the White House telling us, "Aw, y'all don't need to wear a mask," and so people were believing the President of the United States, at the time and in crisis you follow the leader. If there's a fire, you follow the leader ... the person that knows how to get out, that's who we follow. So, we are listening to him, and he has all of these people talking about it's not important to wear the mask, and then we find out that that's wrong. A lot of people suffered ... lost their lives because of that misinformation.

So, I appreciate my pastor who decided – and other pastors like T.D. Jakes – and other pastors of all these megachurches who have the responsibility of thousands in their congregation, and so really does it make sense to tell them, "Your faith is little because you won't bring your people in?" Your twenty-five hundred, three thousand, four thousand to five thousand members in to congregate together and worship together and a whole section of them would end up sick or dead? I don't think that's wisdom, and I don't believe that the God I serve would say that's wisdom. Then not only that, our Word also tells us that we are supposed to follow the laws of the land. So, if we're on lockdown, we're on lockdown. Here's what I love about technology. Here's what I love about the spirit of a Living God: He then gives us this platform – unprecedented – never happened before in our history, that we are now truly, truly the church of God outside of the walls. I know, everybody, whether your church is small or whether you have a megachurch, that's always been something that's been said within the black church, "We're a church that's going outside the walls of this building to serve our community." All right. Well, how about serving the global community now?

I believe God is calling us to one God. He gave me this word back on the Fourth of July: One God. And even this nation that was founded, he reminded me, "One nation. Under God. One God. Indivisible." So, we're already in a problem because we're not focusing under one God, we're not even moving and maneuvering as one nation, and we are for surely not indivisible. Even with this pandemic, even with how the world is right now, as far as the Presidency seat that is open and all the Congress seats that are open right now: we're not indivisible. So, where is this going to land us? As of right now, we're back in another spike. Why? We are divisible. Our divisiveness is really getting ready to kill some people. Yes.

We really have to come as the church of God back *under* God. I do believe that He is begging us to give *us* back to Him. I think of the pandemic of 1918, the Spanish Flu that this has been kind of compared to and did a little research: those people wore masks for over two years. I'm sure there were some skeptics, but back then, if the place is on fire, I'm following who is leading me out of the fire. Wear the mask if that's going to save your life; wear the mask. Why is that an argument? Only because you're hard-headed and don't want to do what you know is right to do, and because you're grown, and you have your own voice, and you can do as you please. But did you ever think about looking at that like murder, so to speak? If you're contagious and you purposely go to work or to the grocery store without your coverings, and you know ... and I won't mention our Commander-in-Chief who has done this very thing – gone in public uncovered with a mask, knowing he had this virus: should he be held responsible for all the people that went to the rallies and caught this virus or to his meetings and caught this virus? For those that have lost their lives, do their families have the right to sue? I don't know ... maybe somebody will call me about that one day; however, I digress. This is about the black church.

Do I think that our church handled this correctly? Yes. I am very appreciative to the leadership of my church -- Omega Baptist Church here in Dayton, Ohio, Senior Pastor Joshua Ward (my shoutout) – how he handled this and he's listening, he believes, to the Word of God that's telling him, "These are your sheep. You are responsible for your sheep." You are responsible for your sheep. You are responsible for your sheep. Your building holds two thousand people? It's not safe per the CDC to have two thousand people gathered at one time. You are responsible for your sheep.

So, thank you to my pastor and all the other leaders around the world that have taken a stance, I believe, under the unction of the Holy Spirit, that say, "Hold on, be still and know that I am God." He also says in the Word that before the Exodus situation in the Bible, and Moses was trying to get everybody free, and all of the plagues came onto the world, what did God say? "Go in your house, but before you go in your house, you anoint your door." Now back then, of course, you had to sacrifice: kill an animal, take the blood, take it around the doorpost. We have Jesus now, so we don't have to do it that way. Just get some oil and anoint your doorpost. Then God says, "Stay put until I tell ya." Now, one thing about the Bible, it does not tell us how long those people were in quarantine. It does not tell us how long that those people were made to stay behind that barrier, if you will, for safety.

We have to get out of our own selves if we truly believe that we are followers of Christ, then we need to start listening to what Christ has to say. I don't think for one minute because He created me that he is going to purposely put us in harm's way. I do have a free will in the decision making on the choice that I make. I'm either going to listen to the Word of God, or I'm going to listen to the word of man.

Black Church: follow the Word of God. We can get through this pandemic with the One that knows how to get us out of it.

That's my take on it. Bye!

HOW I REACHED OUT TO OUR MEMBERS WHEN THE PANDEMIC FORCED OUR CHURCH DOORS TO CLOSE - COVID EXPERIENCE

Dr. Rex al Opusunju

Abounding Love Christian Centre Nigeria Incorporated

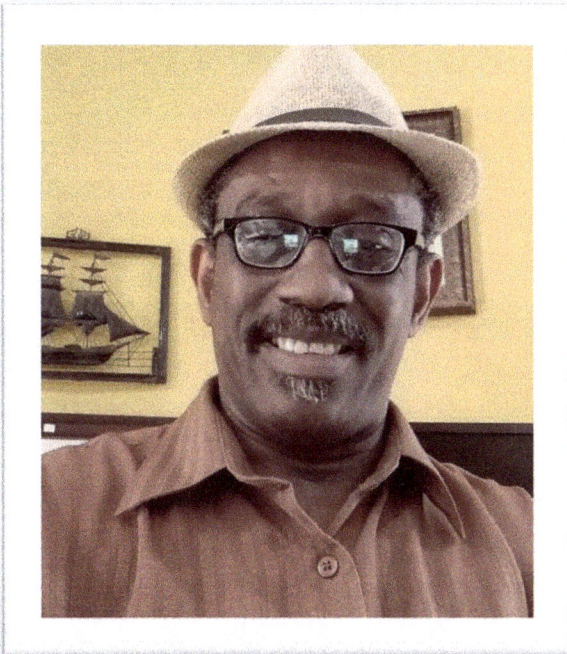

We were able to transition seamlessly during the COVID-19 pandemic lockdown as a church to holding virtual church meetings when it was not possible to meet corporately and physically for worship services and Bible Studies.

Before the COVID-19 pandemic, our ministry had a strong online presence which had spanned for several years. We have several websites with our own domain names and a domain email server. We also have our presence on social media platforms like Facebook and WhatsApp.

During the lockdown I filed an application online for our ministry to use Workplace for Good which is owned by Facebook. Workplace offers corporate organizations the opportunity to connect with their staff remotely using their platform. I was able to set up Workplace for our organization in such a way it reflected the vision of our ministry. First, I had to create email addresses and temporary passwords for the members of our church using our domain email server. Then, I had to invite them to join our organization on Workplace through their email addresses originating from our domain. As soon as they accepted the invitation and joined, holding remote meetings with them on workplace became very easy.

Workplace has the same features with Facebook. I believe Workplace has more superior features than Facebook. I was able to broadcast our meetings on Facebook Live and Workplace Live at the same time. We ran our regular church meetings online.

We had our Bible Studies on Tuesdays, had our Faith Confession Clinic on Wednesdays, held our Prayer meetings on Fridays, and held two worship meetings on Sundays (morning and evening), respectively.

I created about twelve groups on Workplace. We had a prayer group which we populated with our members. We had a Praise and Worship Portal. In this particular portal, I uploaded several inspirational praise and worship videos and songs. Our members could just get in there at their own convenience to listen to several praise and worship songs to build up their faith in God.

We had a group created for children on Workplace. I also took time to upload several Bible stories videos for children in that portal. We had a group created for the youths. I uploaded materials and videos that would teach and inspire the youths to reach their highest potentials in God. I created a group that is an online learning academy for our people to develop several technology skills. We have courses on programming languages like Python. We have full courses on Data Science, SQL, Artificial Intelligence, Machine Learning, Linux, Java, Android, Cyber Security, etc.

We have a group called Faith Hall of Fame. In this group we posted several biographies of men and women God has used beginning with Bible characters like Enoch, Abraham, Noah, and even included several contemporary Christian leaders! The COVID-19 pandemic lockdown has strengthened our capacity as a church to do ministry online.

And this reminds me of the scriptures in Romans 8:28: *And we know that all things work together for good to them that love God, to them who are the called according to his purpose.*

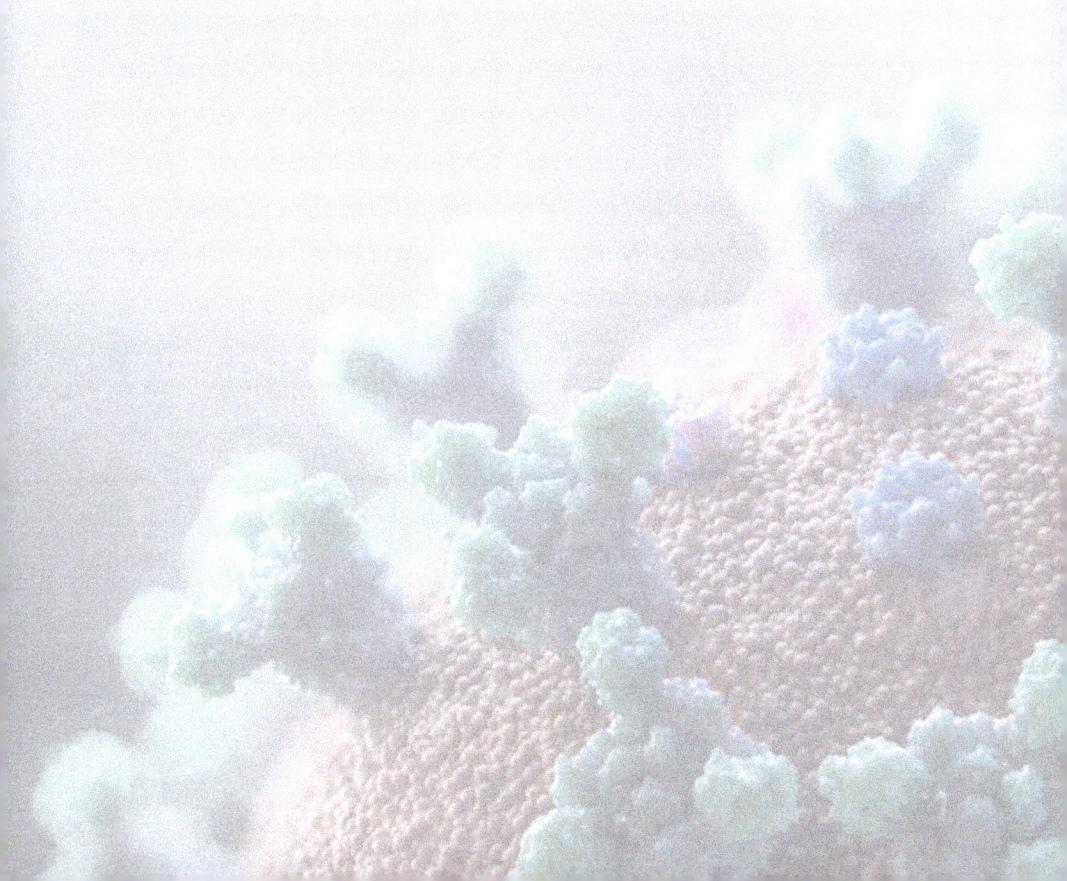

N
ow, let us return to life in the United States of America. During the pandemic there were several local news stories about prisoners catching COVID from staff members. Visitation was cancelled, so the staff members were infecting the prisoners! I began to pray for all prisoners affected and the Lord led me to this scripture in Genesis 40:3 which said:

So he put them in confinement in the house of the captain of the bodyguard, in the jail, the same place where Joseph was imprisoned. This was printed in the New American Standard Bible from: https://bible.knowing-jesus.com/Genesis/40/3

I got excited when I saw the word "confinement" in that scripture, and I was enlightened when I saw the statement "in the house" reflected in that scripture. The *Confinement Chronicles* have been all about various situations that occurred during the pandemic such as mental health, protests, how our children felt, and now, how people received encouragement when gatherings of more than 10 people were cancelled. Pastors had to reach their flock virtually! Teachers had to reach their students virtually, but who did the incarcerated have to reach out to, the staff members that infected them with COVID? Lord, help us!

As I continued to study the word of the Lord with regards to prisoners, I was led to this next scripture in Jeremiah 39:15 – *Now the word of the Lord had come to Jeremiah while he was confined in the court of the guardhouse."* which also came from: https://bible.knowing-jesus.com/topics/Prisoners

This verse led to my greater understanding that, although a person may be confined in a situation, their mind is still open to receiving a word from the Lord! We have all heard stories of prisoners finding salvation while confined. We have heard stories of prisoners learning a trade or even receiving a college degree while incarcerated. These stories are encouraging, yet they should also remind us that PRISONERS NEED THE HELP OF THE CHURCH AFTER THEY ARE RELEASED!

When the doors of the church closed, how were ministry leaders able to reach those released prisoners to help meet THEIR needs? Are we "doing the work of an evangelist" by reaching ALL that may be lost? Some of these released prisoners don't have access to the internet to "Watch the Sunday Service and Wednesday Bible Study". If they couldn't get to your church BEFORE they were locked up, some REALLY don't have a way to log on and watch your live stream! I recently learned that some prisoners don't know how to use a cell phone or set up an email when they are released from prison. You can't send them no "motivational text messages" or emails if they need a lesson on how to use these items. Finally, with the libraries closed during the pandemic, some former prisoners don't even have access to a computer or even a book to read. Did we mail them letters? Did we do a drive-by to leave them a care package or even wave to these former prisoners? What type of encouragement did we offer to prisoners when the Doors of the Church Closed?

This next story was written by a man that found our agency through a family referral. He came to Angie BEE Productions with over seventy hand-written pages ready to be produced into an audiobook. Before we began narration of his project, we decided to ask him a few questions about his life. His words filled my head and my heart, so I asked him to write a segment for *Confinement Chronicles*. The following is what he wrote and how he felt, and it should give an added lesson to the church on how to reach out to the "lost."

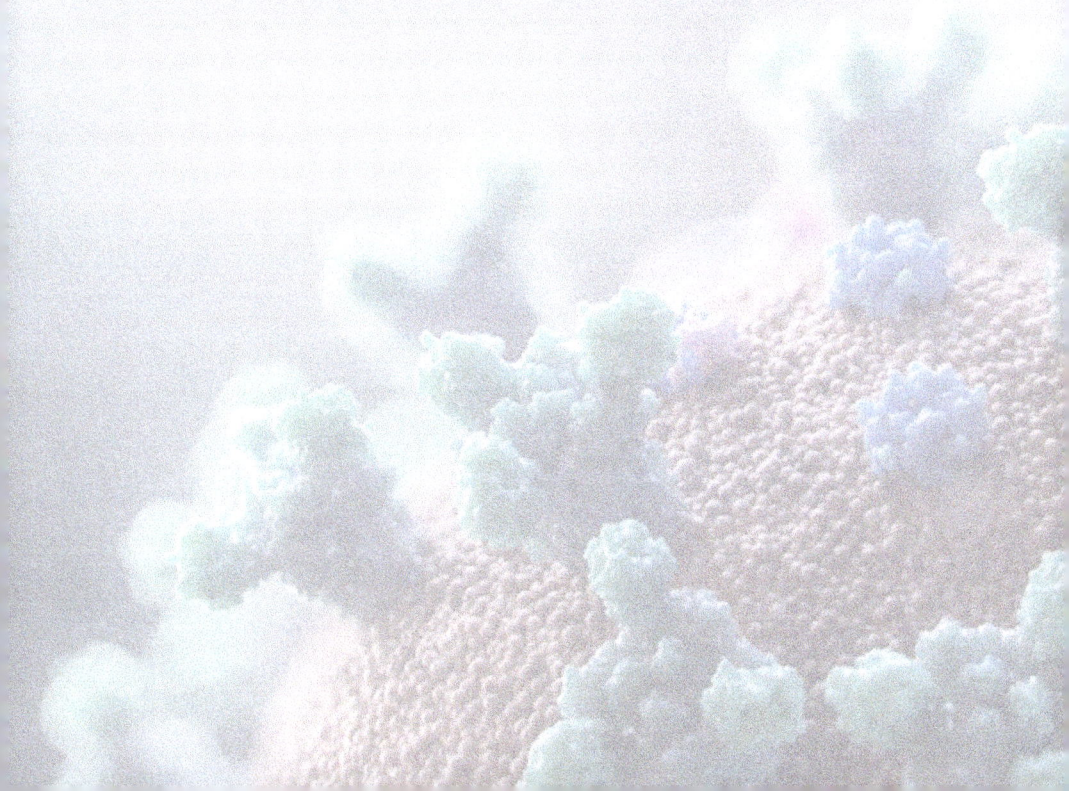

LIFE IN THE PANDEMIC

Ronald Stafford

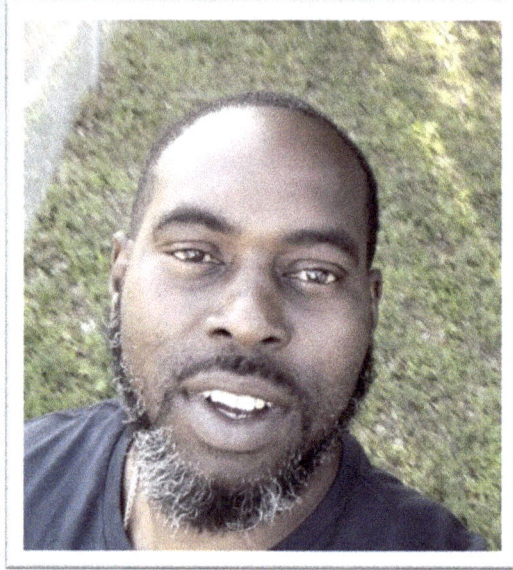

Life in the Pandemic ... it has really been hard, rough, miserable, loss of words, just not right, and WHY? God has His reasons for everything and everybody. Well, since the COVID-19, my life has really changed, but yet just coming back to society, hoping and praying that my life will get better, especially from where I just came.

Five years ago, I came home from prison. Since I got out, I have been searching for jobs, going to interviews, and doing little side-jobs like cutting grass and helping neighbors take out trash. Since COVID hit, I can't do any of those things anymore.

Coming home without not much love or help was even harder, but I tried. Filling out job application after application and hoping for a better start. A lot of work needed; a lot of companies were hiring like construction and road-side assistance, but few will help me to get back to a full-time job. Even friends who could help place me in a job don't seem to be able to help me. Some jobs hiring and some "got their picks."

Well, sitting back waiting for a call – HELL – something got to give! I still have needs and wants but can't reach them. Don't want to go back to what I know, but HELL; I might not have a choice.

NO CHOICE!

Family and few friends helping me out, but how long will that last? They are having trouble in this pandemic, too. When will this all end?

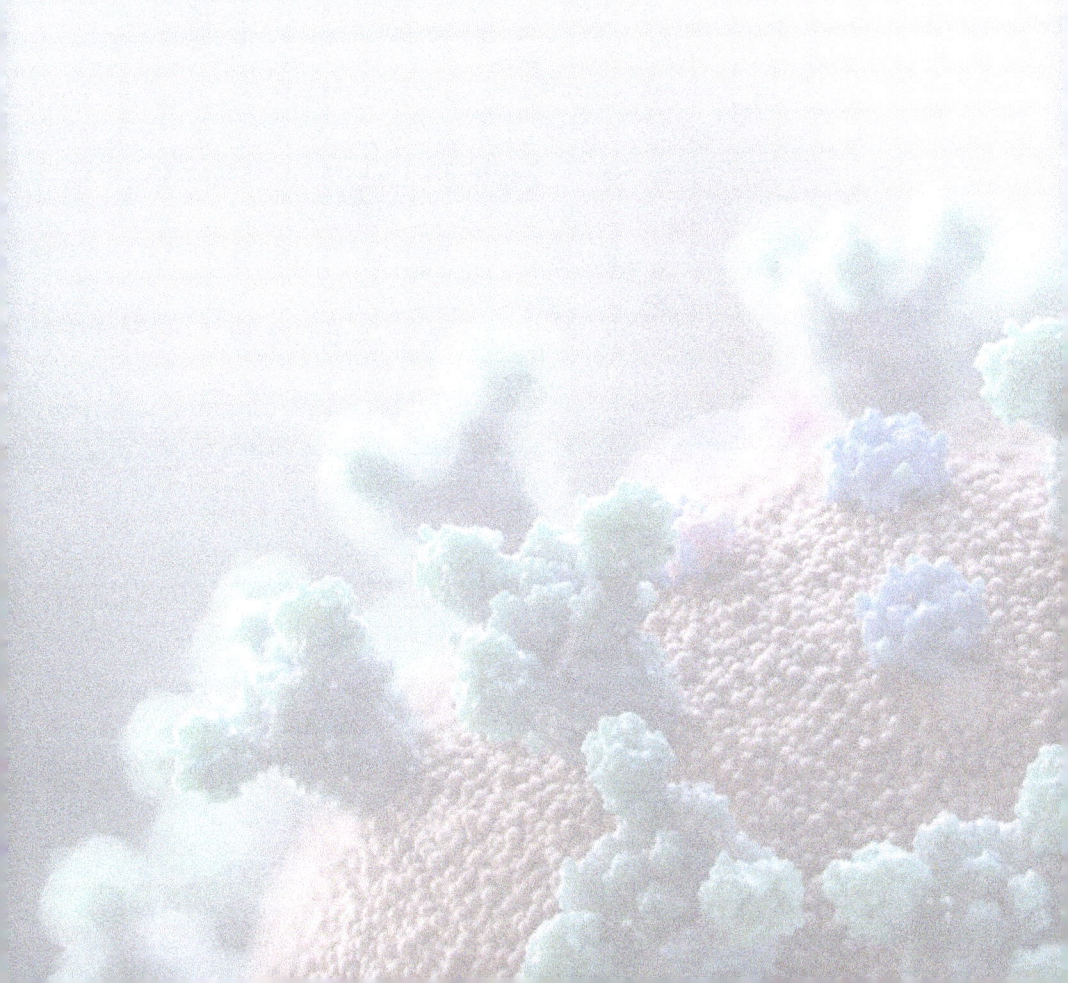

URBAN YOUTH JUSTICE, INC.

Our Story

Pedro Rodriguez

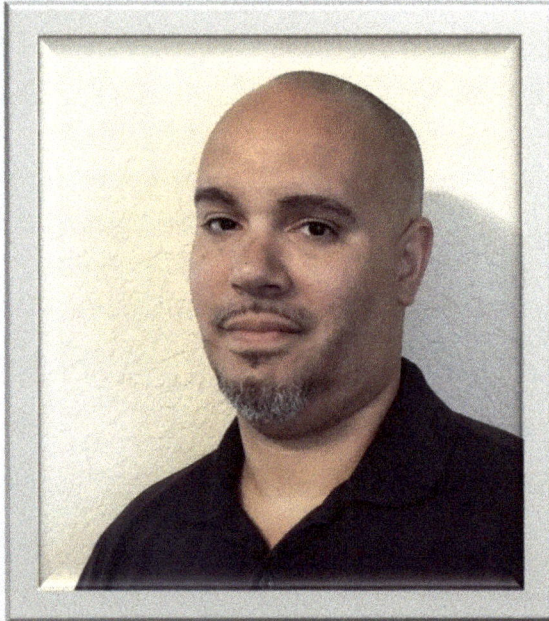

Pedro and Gedia Rodriguez are the founders of Urban Youth Justice, Inc. The two have been married for twenty-one years and are parents to five adult children. Both grew up fatherless, and as a result, experienced much pain and suffering growing up in single parent homes. Their relationship revealed how much they were missing something. They later discovered it was God they were missing, and they decided to marry, and together, they pursued a relationship with Christ.

After coming to Christ, they connected with a local church where they grew and became leaders. They still had many obstacles to overcome, but they were determined to do life together and discover their calling. About sixteen years later, they were seeking guidance on their next move, and the Lord presented them an opportunity to move to Florida. The first few years, they struggled to find their place in the West Bradenton neighborhood. They began to ask God what it was that He wanted them to do in this community.

They began to see God move and open doors for ministry. Pedro knew God was calling him to do prison ministry but did not know where to start. He began a journey to network and meet people who could guide him in the right direction. After years of volunteering with a few different organizations such as Prison Fellowship and Youth for Christ, he knew God was leading him to start his own nonprofit organization. He and his wife had been doing juvenile justice ministry a few years before they decided to launch Urban Youth Justice.

U.Y.J. was launched in 2019, and it rapidly expanded. This organization was created to meet the needs of fatherless and justice-involved youth. There are so many youths who fall under this demographic; there is much work to be done. They prayed for the Lord to help them build a team, and God answered their prayer. They now have over twenty different men and women who have joined them on this mission to reach justice involved youth throughout the state of Florida. Over the past year, they have received support, resources, and financial contributions to carry out their mission. Some of the organizations and churches that have supported them include Tampa Underground, St. Pete Underground, Every Youth Every Facility, Grace Life Church, and Harbor Community Church.

Within this first year of doing ministry as a nonprofit, an unexpected state of emergency, known as the COVID-19 pandemic, put a temporary halt to their ministry. Their ministry consisted of going into several facilities in a few counties and sharing the gospel with the youth who were currently detained. They do this by using Christian Hip Hop, teaching life skills, and mentoring youth upon release. Not being able to go in physically caused them to think outside the box and use technology as the method of delivery. They began to record music, personal stories, and a biblical message on DVDs and delivered them to all the facilities they serve. U.Y.J. was able to partner with 4th Purpose Foundation who created a series of videos called "Visitation 2.0" for those who were incarcerated. U.Y.J. was able to deliver these videos to hundreds of youths at several facilities. After a few months, they also began to use Zoom as a method of communication with the youth inside the facilities. Their ministry team also used this form of communication to stay connected and have a time of prayer for the youth inside and for one another. Just recently, they launched a podcast called *Voices of Truth* which gives a voice to those who do urban missions in the detention centers or their local urban community. The podcast was created as a resource to reach youth but also to encourage people to join the mission. This is one of several things the Lord has allowed them to do during this challenging time. It has been an interesting year but one that has still shown to produce great outcomes.

Throughout this first year, they were able to launch their website UYJINC.org and become a 501c3 nonprofit organization. Urban Youth Justice did not allow the pandemic to stop them. They continued to endure the challenges and persist on the journey to reach the youth. Many of these youths could not receive visits from family or volunteers, but Urban Youth Justice has made it their mission to reach hundreds of youths in ten facilities across six counties in Florida so far. We have now been able to go back into the facilities with the safety requirements in place, and the youth were excited to see us and were encouraged by the hope and love we bring to these facilities.

There are still some facilities we have not been able to enter but are still using technology to reach them while we also pray for them and the staff that work with them. We know that COVID-19 is long from gone but instead of allowing it to shut us down, it motivated us to find new and fresh ways to accomplish what God has called us to do. We are grateful for every opportunity we get to enter these facilities with the goal to bring justice and restore hope to a young fatherless generation.

God has continued to be at work in their ministry even throughout the pandemic. Join us in praying that He would continue to guide them and provide for them in their mission!

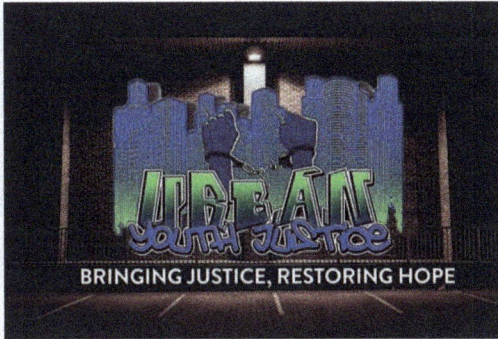

BRINGING JUSTICE, RESTORING HOPE

Lord, I see what you are doing in this season. People couldn't get IN to the church, because the doors were closed, so the church came to the people! As I was reflecting upon these stories, the Spirit of the Lord led me to another scripture. Some of us are quite familiar with the verse: *You have not because you ask not*, but have you ever read the ENTIRE passage from James 4:2-3? Well, here ya go – I will read it to you:

> *You desire but do not have, so you kill. You covet but you cannot get what you want, so you quarrel and fight. You do not have because you do not ask God. ³ When you ask, you do not receive, because you ask with wrong motives, that you may spend what you get on your pleasures.*
> James 4:2-3 (New International Version)

As evangelists and servants of the Lord, we have been charged with bringing the Gospel of Jesus Christ to the lost and the down-trodden. If you ever needed a blueprint to accomplish this task, James 4: 2-3 illuminates the way for us.

You desire but do not have, so you kill.

Let us reach others to teach them how to fill those desires. Let us feed them, clothe them, house them, and employ them to give them a hope! Then their eyes will be open to the grace and mercy of God.

You covet but you cannot get what you want, so you quarrel and fight.

Let us reach others to help them see the blessings that they currently have: life, health, strength and hope! Not necessarily to remain in a pit of despair, but to use this appreciation to give God glory! Quarrel and fighting during this pandemic could end if we could all appreciate rather than covet.

You do not have because you do not ask God. ³ When you ask, you do not receive, because you ask with wrong intentions, wrong motives, that you may spend what you get on your pleasures.

Let us continue to reach others and encourage them to *Look to the hills from which cometh their health and strength,* yet to do so with a humble nature, not with greed in their hearts.

Think about a small child asking their parents for a cookie. We are the child asking Our Father for something that we "want", but not necessarily for something that we "need." God will not grant us our "wishes" because that request is to satisfy our "pleasures." God will give us what we need and even more than we could ask or even think about! Let us reach others with this good news! Let us "do the work of an evangelist" and give God praise as we do it!

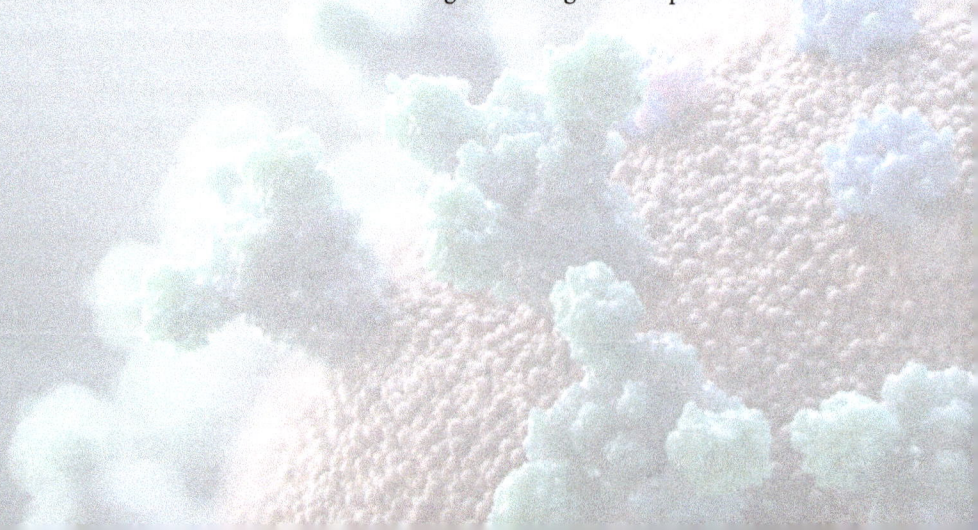

... AND THE BAND PLAYED ON

Sonya Bennett

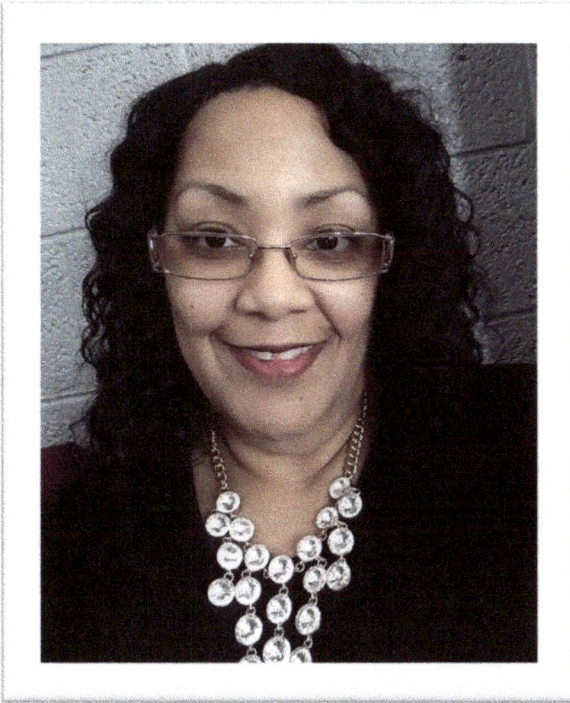

For as long as I can remember, music has been a part of my life: 45s spinning on the record player while we cleaned up on Saturday mornings, learning to play the violin in third grade, singing in the Cherubic, Young Adult, Mumford High School Choirs, and the list goes on and on. My father is a singer; my sister is a former pianist; my mother loved dancing; and one sister is a cellist – music has always surrounded me. I think of the Titanic, and as the ship's occupants were evacuating (according to the movie), the band played on. In the midst of this pandemic, I think of that tenacity and dedication as seemingly everything around us is deteriorating.

March 2020: my pastor, under Executive Order of the Governor, followed the arduous decision that the physical services of Beth Eden Missionary Baptist Church would cease and go virtual. It had been less than a year that I was invited to minister with our Praise Team: a condensed version of our music ministry. Initially, I declined – setting the atmosphere of praise is entirely different than combining voices with tenors, altos, and sopranos of a choir because of the intensity of a smaller group. I spoke with my father who reminded me that this is an honor and one that shouldn't be taken lightly. Then the pandemic happened, and the responsibility has increased: I STILL get nervous as we prepare to minister, even virtually. I went from breaking speed limits to arrive at church on time on Sunday mornings to gathering in our empty sanctuary with our Quarantine Crew to practice and record our church services. In these months, many have complained that they are "ready" to congregate physically, missing the normalcy of church; however, I always reply that God has never been normal.

Just singing to an empty sanctuary is rough. I don't know how to end this story because it is still going on.

You may watch our Sunday services each week online at
www.BEedenNation.com

. . . The band played on.

THE CHURCH IN THE COVID-19 PANDEMIC

Pastor Patrick Wilkerson

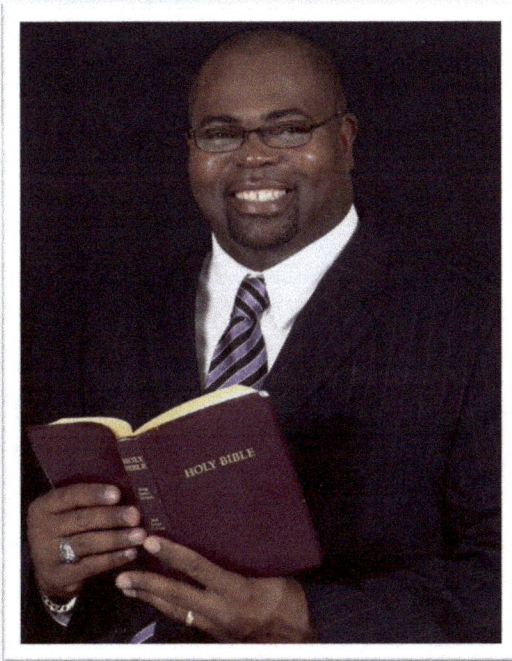

In December of 2019, the COVID-19 Pandemic had started to affect our society. The information that was being put out by our government officials was slanted for political reasons. The Christian Members of the body of Christ continued to lean more on their faith than the altered/inaccurate medical information that was given.

When the New Year 2020 arrived, the church started to see a decline in the personal attendance and fellowship, due to the fact that COVID-19 pandemic numbers continued to increase. In March of 2020, the personal attendance came to a shocking halt, due to the number of deaths and severe sickness from COVID-19. Many church members were very emotionally stressed about not being able to attend church together. Many members expressed they had never experienced the church doors being closed for any reasons. The church building was where they could come to pray, fellowship with family and friends, and gain strength and encouragement from powerful preached sermons. The one place they had to come and get some hope was now closed. Both the old and young people expressed the same hurts and disappointment. I, as the Pastor, must continually encourage the people of God, that "God is in control" and that God is with us "for such a time as this." I continue to teach and preach the Word of God through Bible lessons and sermons to inform the body of Christ that "this too shall pass." My personal prayers to God were accentuated, to include God's desire for our local church.

I received spiritual confirmation to execute "Sunday Morning Drive-In Worship Service" in Flagler County and stream live on Facebook weekly. There is a drive-in church in Daytona Beach Shores that has operated for many years. God used them as a model for what I should do for my parishioners. When I presented my desire to the church ministry leaders, it was received and embraced positively. We began our "Drive-In Worship Service" in April 2020. The church members and local community responded very well. The worship services were uplifting, we all had a chance to see each other. We wore masks and practiced social distancing, as required. We could not get out of our cars to greet or hug each other, but we were able to talk, share smiles, share affectionate gestures, and wave to each other. We continued the Drive-In Worship Service every Sunday morning until June 2020, when the daily high very hot temperatures in Florida began to affect the comfort level of those attending. The temperature was becoming unbearable, and some members stopped attending for that reason. The COVID-19 illnesses and deaths continued to rise. Several members within the congregation were diagnosed positive with COVID-19, and some were hospitalized for several days. We thank God for his healing grace because each member has recovered and is doing well. Some type of service continued into June, but due to the weather and more members testing positive for COVID, we had to pause.

Our youth members were disappointed and confused, but so was I as their pastor. So now, we have moved to streaming live on Facebook from my home; everything and everyone is on lockdown because of the pandemic. Many of our senior members did not know how to go to view the services livestream. We had several members that volunteered to go to the homes and give training and instructions on viewing worship service online streaming.

They learned well and are even having Virtual Worship Watch Parties. The older and younger members are also giving their financial tithes and offerings electronically and online. God is so good. One of my favorite verses in the Bible, Isaiah 40:8 says, *"The grass withereth, flower fadeth: but the word of our God shall stand forever."*

During this pandemic, the church body has been encouraged to stand on the Word of God and follow the medical professionals' instructions. As of the date of this writing, our local church continues to livestream from the church sanctuary with limited in attendance. Yes, we all miss the fellowship, but we do have conference call meetings and ZOOM Fellowship events. Our youth, toddlers, and school age children, they miss running and playing with each other. To keep our young people engaged in the ministry, we continue to be creative. I, as their pastor, engage weekly with them on ZOOM Virtual Fellowship to discuss the issues of the day, answer any questions regarding news, politics or community concerns and keep them engaged in the ministry.

One youth event was a VIRTUAL ZOOM "Cooking with Mrs. Queen" from South Carolina and "Cooking with Pastor P." The youth had a great time: they each made peach cobbler pies and homemade biscuits for their individual homes. In my opinion, this pandemic has done two things: it has brought out the best and the worst in people. I clearly understand that I cannot follow what my other clergy friends will or will not do; I must follow as God directs me for this local ministry that I lead and pastor. As I continue to pray without ceasing for spiritual direction, I will continue to follow God's prompting and also adhere to the medical professional advice for the safety and well-being of the members. I will continue to encourage the members to be obedient to God and to do so without complaining.

This concludes *Confinement Chronicles*, Volume VI

As we now end, we encourage you to order Volumes I, II, III and IV and the entire 10 – volume series! Place your order and follow **Confinement Chronicles by Angie BEE Productions on Facebook**. As this series grows, we pray that you share them with others, and learn from them as well.

These stories shall continue!

Be safe and BEE Blessed
Sincerely,
Evangelist Angie BEE

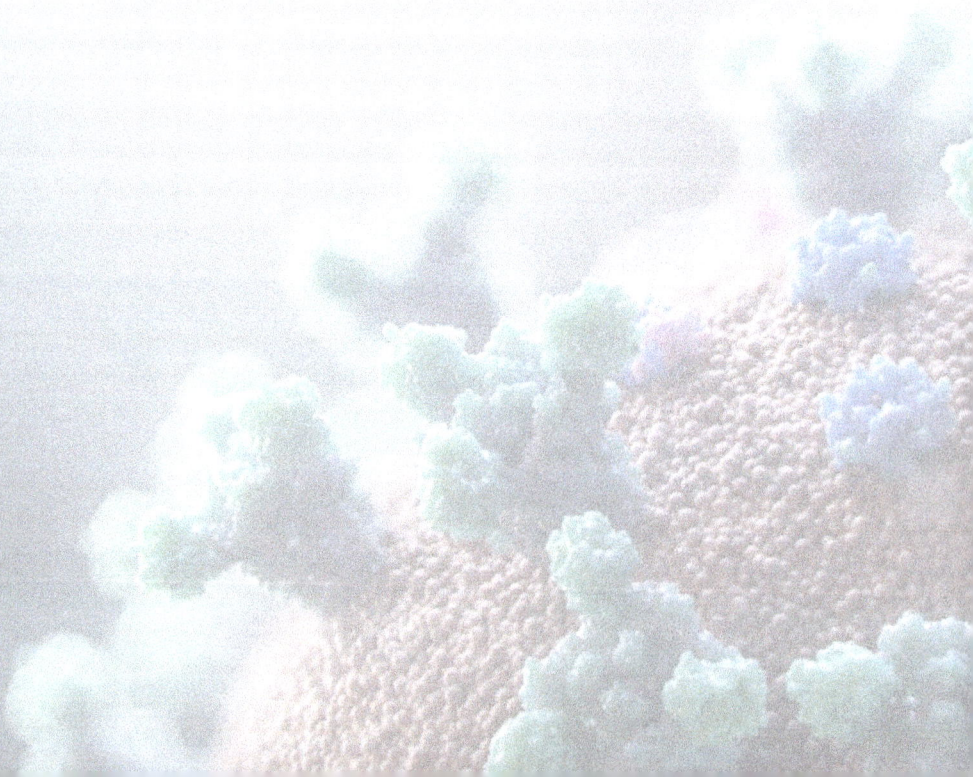

VOLUME VII

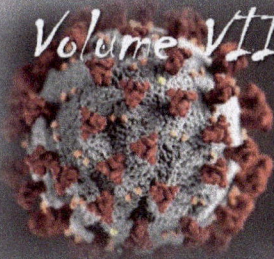

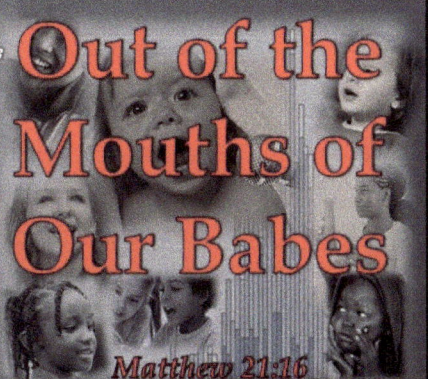

Confinement Chronicles
Pandemic Stories from Our Children

Volume VII

Out of the Mouths of Our Babes

Matthew 21:16

An inspirational audiobook compilation series produced by

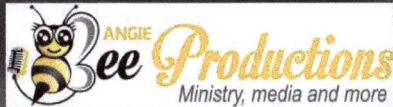

ANGIE Bee Productions
Ministry, media and more

W e have arrived at Volume VII, and it is time to hear from our babies, the young people who were affected by this pandemic. They had to learn to attend school from home; they had to learn to wear a mask; they missed their friends, and now they are sharing their stories . . .

And now, for our first contribution . . .

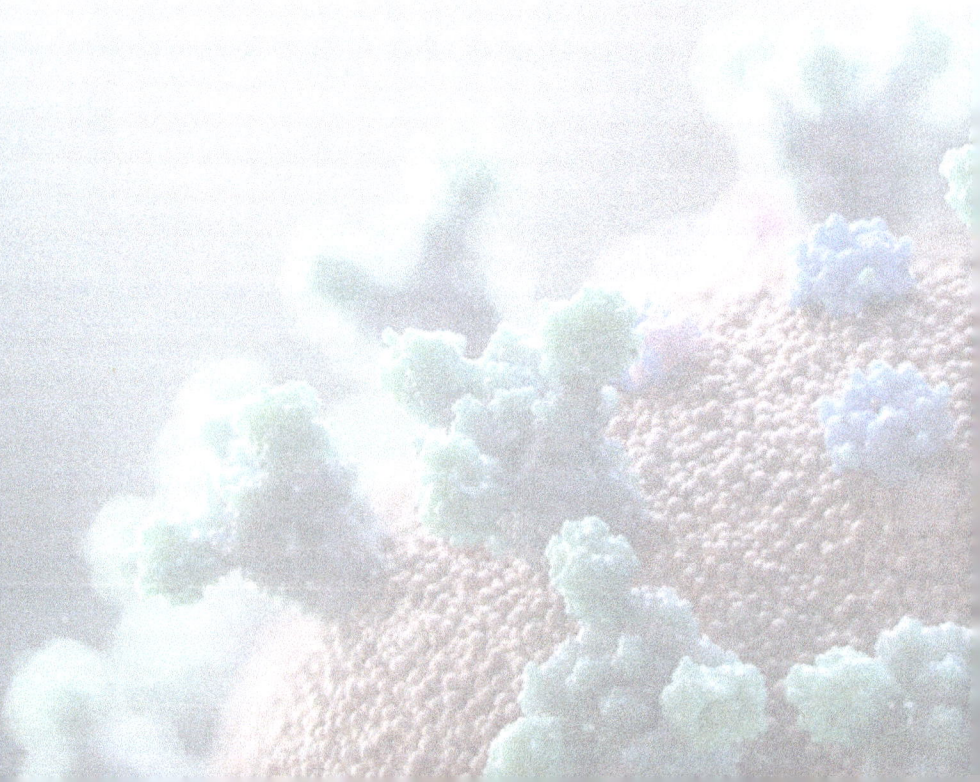

MY FEELINGS ABOUT THIS PANDEMIC

Kami Love

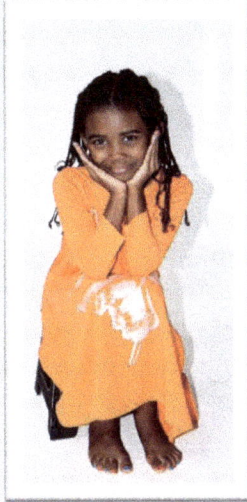

Good Day, everyone. I am Kami Love. I am here to talk about my pandemic experience.

The pandemic has been hard on me because I was stuck inside with no video games and no friends. My parents were the only friends that I have while social distancing. I miss my school friends a lot. I will not be returning to traditional school in the fall, instead virtual school again. I will really miss all of my friends. It has been very boring to stay in the house. We recently moved during the pandemic, and my parents bought me a blow-up pool. I have enjoyed being able to swim and splash in my backyard. We have a bunch of boards games to play with. The pandemic has allowed me and my parents to become closer.

This pandemic has ruined my chance to see my best friend who is out of state. We are not able to go on vacation or out of town. We are not able to enjoy the amazing amusement parks here in Florida.

The pandemic was also hard on my friendships. I will not be able to see my friends until the pandemic ends which may not be until 2021. I hope that it isn't that long. I don't like the coronavirus, because it came out of nowhere in the middle of March, right after my birthday. Now, the laws have changed to where everyone is social distancing, having to stay away six feet. You have to wear a mask everywhere: through which is hot and hard to breathe.

People are losing their lives to the virus and getting very sick. The test is expensive to be tested and takes a long time to come back to tell you if you are sick or not. I just want the Pandemic to END!

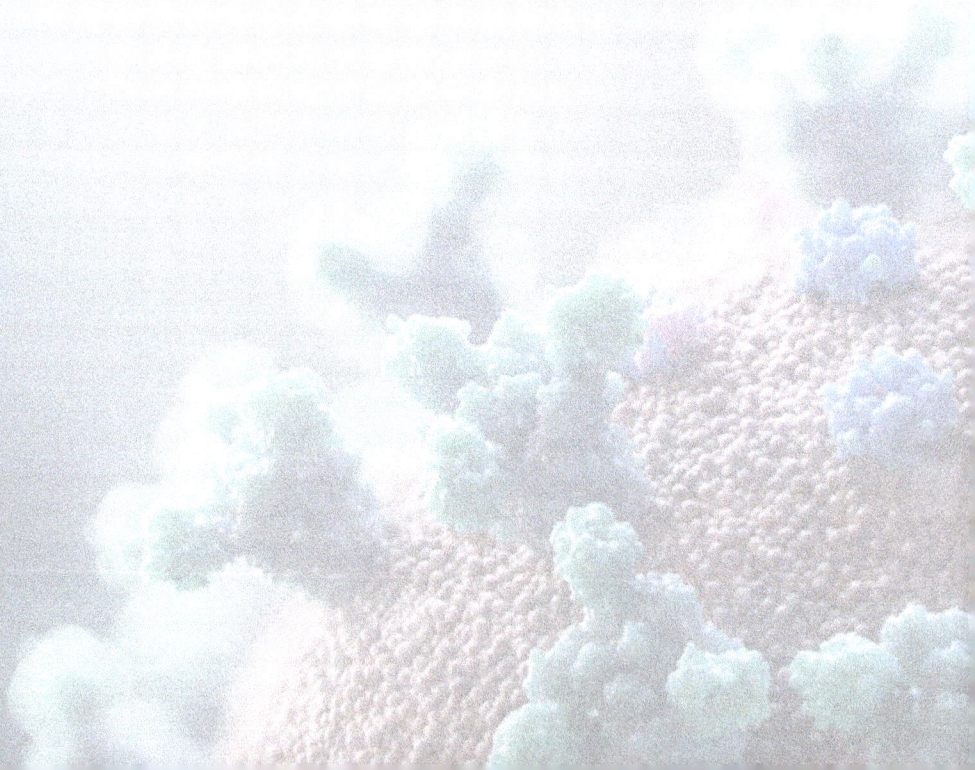

My Time Looking for Toilet Paper

Jalen Alexander

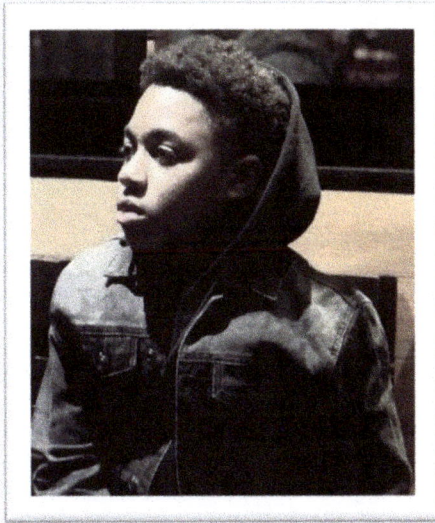

Hi, my name is Jalen Spicer. I'm fifteen years old and in the 10th grade. Quarantine: that's the subject for today or has been for a while now. Let me start from the beginning. Before quarantine, I was at school, just a regular day but not fully at its state of normality, as everyone was talking about the virus either as a joke, seriously, or just didn't speak about it at all. There was a great mixture of these people as we talked about the Virus. We would think about the ups and downs of having no school as there would be no work, but we may have summer school, but I don't think any of us expected THIS. Slowly but surely, schools are starting to close down. My school gets closed. At first, I didn't see it as a huge thing; I just thought we're going to go back. But we didn't; online classes were in order. When they started, I was worried about keeping up with my work. I've always been bad with online work. But when I found out doing the work wasn't mandatory, I didn't take it seriously. My family tried to get me to stay consistent. It failed. What has kept my time occupied is the constant thoughts of things I could do. New skills, so many ideas! I always end up just playing video games. Overall, quarantine has been perfectly fine to me. I'm fine with staying in the house. I'm ok with going outside for a second and coming right back in. I don't mind this. This is life now. I've adapted.

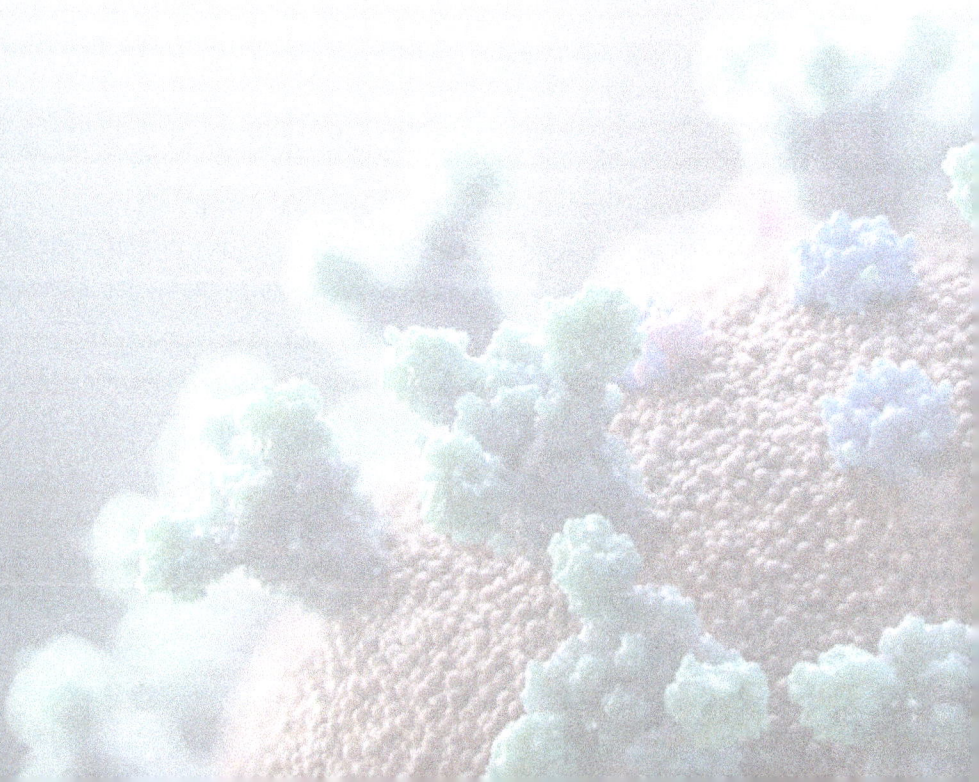

Out of the Mouth of Babes

Theresa Jordan

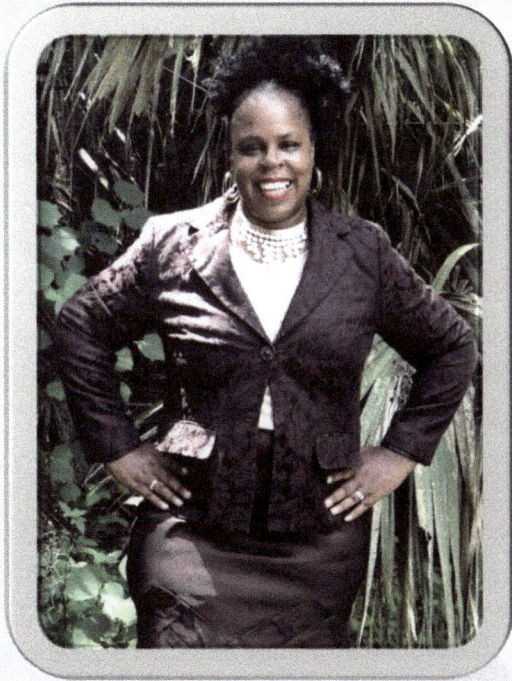

I am sitting here contemplating how excellent God is and how marvelous His ways are toward us. I begin to get overwhelmed by God's love, mercy, grace, and faithfulness toward all of us every day. I am constantly reminded that God's ways are not like our ways, and His Word is relevant in the times we are facing right now. I am reminded His Word is the same yesterday, today and forevermore. I am profound because, *"Out of the mouth of babes and sucklings hast thou ordained strength."* (Psalm 8:2). During these unprecedented times, I have witnessed children between the ages of 4 months to 16 years old declaring and decreeing God's word throughout this pandemic to the entire world. These captivating videos shared through Facebook and several other platforms will be a treasure for me for the rest of my life. The Bible says, *"Train up a child in the way he should go: and when he is old, he will not depart from it."* (Proverbs

22:6). I have watched several videos showing these pure conversations that were coming out of the mouths of our children.

One video was when three young girls were having church at home during this quarantine, and one of the girls was the preacher and she converted a chair to a pulpit. This was astonishing to see, especially because of her youth. She knew how to improvise even at a young age, and she knew how to make things work. Apparently, the congregation consisted of her two siblings, and they were girls close to her age. The two girls were sitting on their toys, and the third little girl was reading a book. The book she had on her pulpit represented the Bible, and she proceeded to open her bible. She brought forth the word, and she wanted the congregation and the world to know that God can do everything. She made it clear how much she loved the Lord. This baby proceeded to speak, and she ended her service singing this song, "Oh, I came to tell you what Jesus said, He said repent of your sins and be baptized." This was an exceeding and spectacular moment for me; it left me flabbergasted again because this was coming forth out of the mouth of babes.

Another incident is about a young man who captured my heart because he was giving his grandmother recognition in front of the world. This sincerely touched my heart because he was giving his grandmother her flowers while she was living. He was willing to give his grandmother an opportunity to smell her flowers by hearing every single word he had to say to his grandmother. She did not have to wait to be celebrated when she could not hear these profound words during her celebration of life. Therefore, this third video was a climax for me because the grandson came outside of the house, and if I were to speculate, I believe he was in front of his grandmother's house. He took the time to acknowledge and encourage his grandmother first, and then he continued to encourage the world with the Word of God. This young man opened by saying, "Your past does not determine your future." He proceeded to say, "Your condition is not your conclusion." He wanted everyone to know we served the true and living God, and He is our Alpha & Omega. He wanted to encourage everyone to hold unto God's unchanging hands, and that God is able to make a way out of no way.

Everything I have experienced throughout these past months has made me more appreciative of God's faithfulness, and it has been so fulfilling to watch our youth boldly and confidently proclaim the Word of God. God's promises have been manifested in the lives of our youth, and this should serve as a confirmation that "God will do, what He said He would do." This should also serve as evidence hearing our children come forth and declare the Word of God.

Experiencing all of this brings me to several of my favorite songs, "God is Faithful to Perform His Word" by Norman Hutchins. Here are some of the words to the song: *God is bigger than my mountain. Bigger than my valley, Bigger than my headache, and he is bigger than my pain.* It is a constant reminder that God is faithful!

The next song is "Great is Thy Faithfulness" by Pastor Donnie McClurkin. This resonates with me because God is faithful toward all of us every day.

God's Word says, *Be careful for nothing; but in everything by prayer and supplication with thanksgiving let your requests be made known unto God.* (Philippians 4:6).

We can take it a step further by declaring and decreeing what the Lord has already spoken, *For I know the thoughts that I think toward you, saith the Lord, thoughts of peace, and not of evil, to give you an expected end.* (Jeremiah 29:11).

My hope is that these highlighted and fascinating stories will inspire you to keep your faith, and they will also help you to realize "This battle is not yours, it is the Lord's" by Yolanda Adams. My hope is that you will always be encouraged in the Lord and that you will continue standing on the promises of God.

A FUTURE IS SOMETHING I DESIRE

Dion Taylor

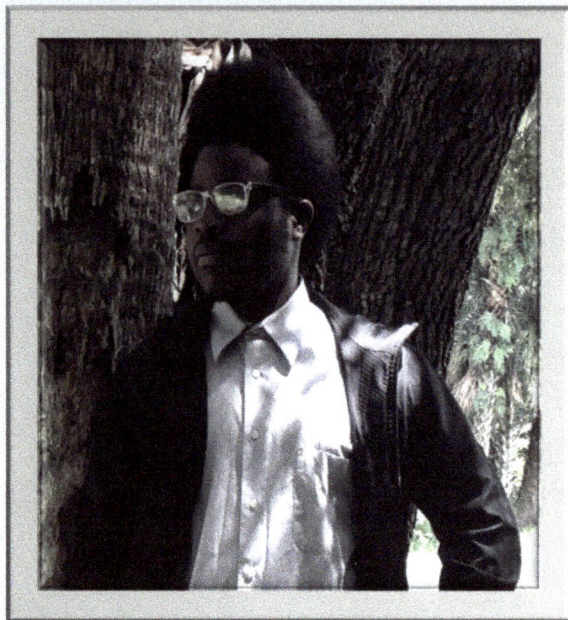

The times we may be going through right now are not to our liking, but we will get through it. I am sure during these times we all have done some thinking. As much as I would say I did not like school, but now I sort of miss it – not the schoolwork, but the people that came with it. I moved to Florida a couple years ago, and then I moved back to New Jersey. I recently moved back in November 2019, so the time feels so short. I have been making new friends and going to new places, and this was something I was starting to get used to. There were some things that I took for granted – especially, realizing the changes that came with this pandemic. They are not exactly what everyone wants, but it is what we need for now. That makes me wonder how life will be after all of this is over with, and the changes that will come with this new life. I doubt it will be the same, and we will have to find a new "normal." Even with all of that said, this pandemic has given me a lot of time to think about myself and my future. I also realized that everyone is not exactly helping the situation. Some are willing to wear masks and practice social distancing, while others are just saying, "whatever" or "I don't need to" and some are throwing parties. I will never understand some of these people. A future is something I desire very much, so I will do what I can for the others around me and myself. That is because many families' loved ones are gone, and that is never exactly easy to get over. I am familiar with that all too well myself. This pandemic has had many positive and negative effects on me and others around the world. I have come to the realization that life is always what it has been . . . "fragile."

All of us are so busy with our lives that we forget to think. That is what this quarantine has given me, and there is no way I wasn't going to take advantage of it.

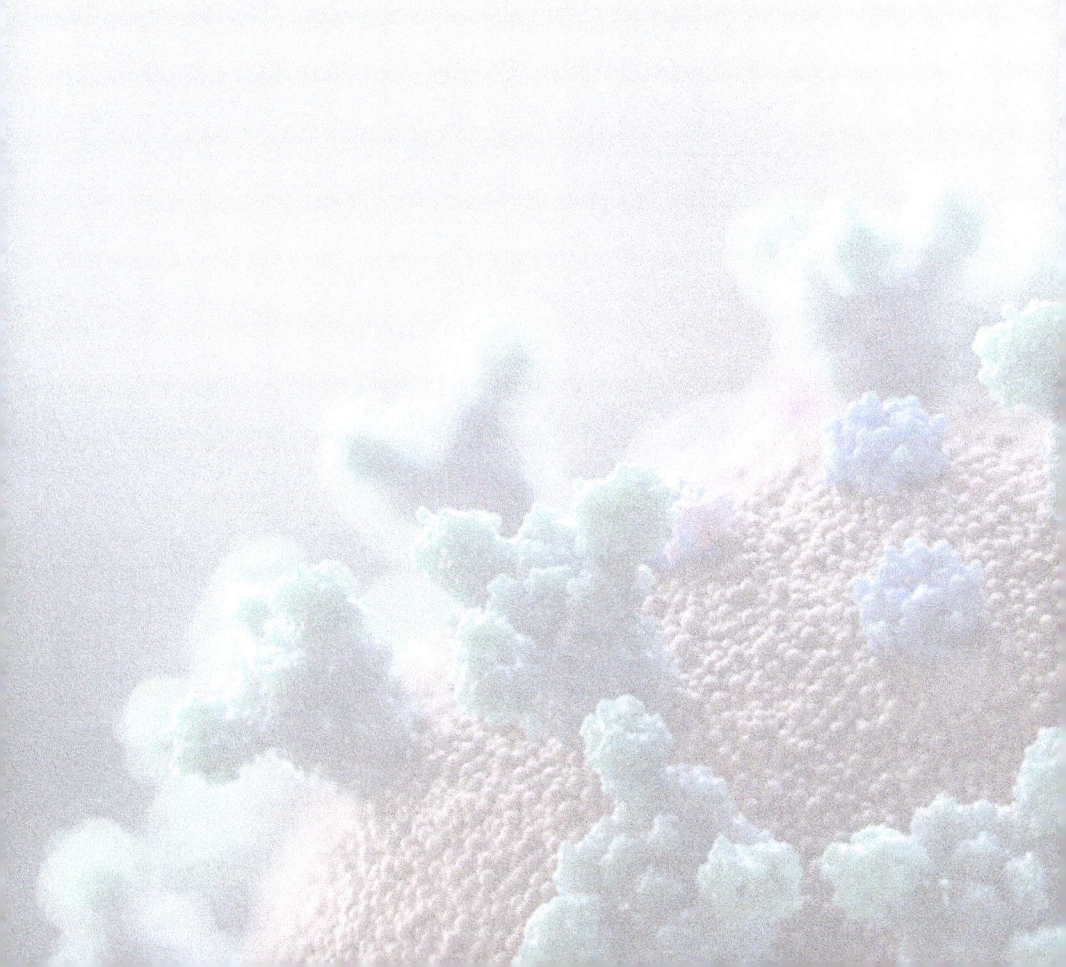

AN INTIMATE CONVERSATION

Between Evangelist Angie BEE & Her Niece Sandra "Bee"

Angie BEE: Okay, Sandra, tell me: how do you feel about the coronavirus?

Sandra: I hate it because the Governor keeps putting extra days that we have to stay in quarantine, and I want to go out and play and go back to school. When I was still in school, I wanted to NOT go to school some days, and now all I want to do is go to school. It's boring at home: If you're an only child with just a mother here, then it's boring at home.

Angie BEE: I understand. So, tell me: what is the coronavirus?

Sandra: It's a little ball with things sticking out of it.

Angie BEE: That's what the picture looks like?

Sandra: Yeah!

Angie BEE: What else do you know about the coronavirus?

Sandra: It's spreading nationwide.

Angie BEE: What does "nationwide:" mean?

Sandra: The whole world.

Angie BEE: So, it's spreading globally. The whole world? Are you scared?

Sandra: No.

Angie BEE: Why not?

Sandra: It's not scary because if you've gotten tested and you don't have it, then there's a 0000.1% chance of you getting it. And if you already have it, there is a 1000% chance that you will survive it.

Angie BEE: Do you know anyone who has survived it?

Sandra: Yes.

Angie BEE BEE: How does that make you feel?

Sandra: I'm surprised that he survived it!

Angie BEE: Why?

Sandra: Because he had a bunch of things. He had pneumonia, the flu, and coronavirus. All the people who had coronavirus died, but he had more things than they had, and he still survived.

Angie BEE: That's good. So how do you feel about your friends in the middle of the coronavirus? Do you worry about them? Do you think they're safe?

Sandra: No. I don't worry about them that much. I don't worry that they're not safe because I know they're safe because they live in neighborhoods that are safe, nothing happens, no one has the virus.

Angie BEE: Okay. Do you worry about your mom? She has to go outside and risk being exposed to the virus to take you places, get groceries, and to get the things you need. Do you worry about her?

Sandra: No. For her 51st birthday, I'm going to buy her a hazmat suit.

Angie BEE: Okay. But what about today, do you worry?

Sandra: No.

Angie BEE: Okay. What about your family that lives in other places? Do you worry about them?

Sandra: No.

Angie BEE: So, you're not worried about coronavirus at all? That's good! Why do you think that you have so much faith and you're not worried?

Sandra: We're safe. What's faith?

Angie BEE: What does your shirt say?

Sandra: I can't read it… (Sandra's mother says – *it's upside down*… "Faith Over Fear") Faith Over Fear

Angie BEE: So, you're not worried about people because you have *Faith Over Fear*. Do you know what that means?

Sandra: No.

Angie BEE: Faith means that you believe in God, and you believe that God is going to take care of things, so you don't worry about your mommy and your friends; you just don't worry because you know that God is going to take care of it. "Faith NO Fear" means that you're not afraid of nothing. Right?!

Sandra: Okay.

Angie BEE: Would you like to add anything else as we complete this interview about the coronavirus? What else would you like to tell me? I am listening!

Sandra: Yes. Sometimes people always go out and Mommy sees them in the store, and they don't have a mask, they don't have a hazmat suit. They don't have anything to protect them from the virus.

Angie BEE: And how do you feel about that?

Sandra: I want to tell them to put on a mask! Put on gloves! Put on a hazmat suit; just don't get the virus because if you come back here and give me the virus, I'm beating you up when I survive!

Angie BEE: Oh, Lord! Well, may I make a suggestion? Maybe, instead of saying those things to them – because sometimes, it's just inappropriate to say certain things to grown-ups ...

Sandra: I never say those things. I just say them in my head ...

Angie BEE: I gotcha! What else can you say in your head?

Sandra: People need to stop smoking and loitering.

Angie BEE: Yeah, that's true. The other thing you could say in your head is, "Jesus, please protect them"; you could pray over them.

Sandra: Yeah.

Angie BEE: Okay, thank you for this time, I appreciate your input. I love you. My Baby!! Gimme that nose and cheek and other cheek (kiss kiss).

Sandra: IT TICKLES!

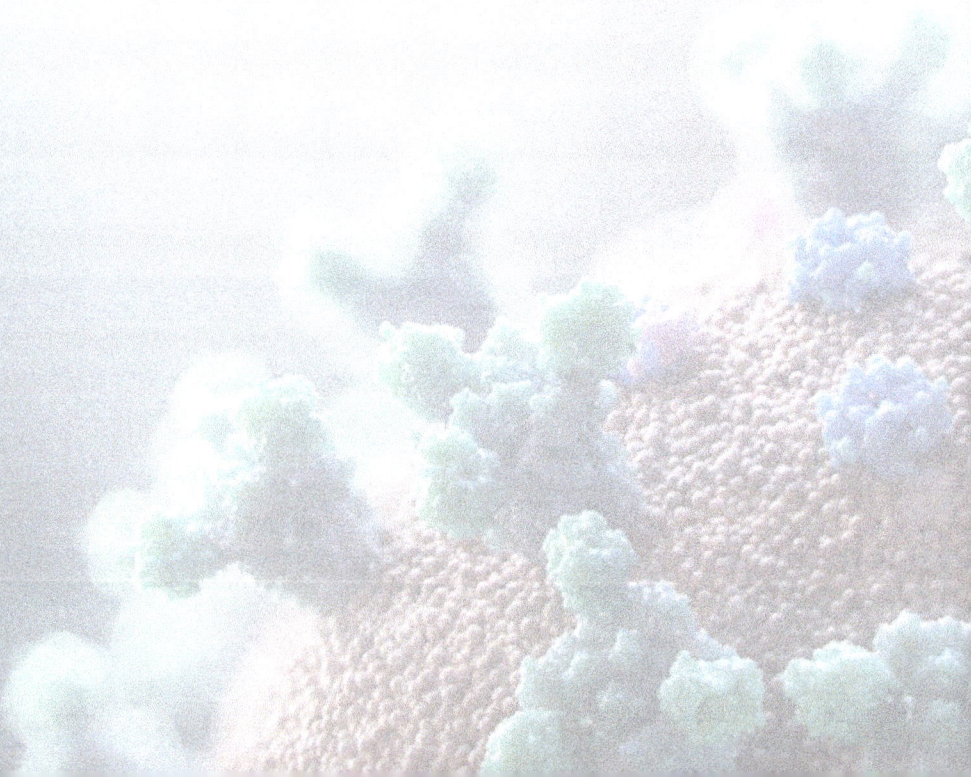

During this pandemic, I have been inspired and encouraged by several young people around me. I watched the newlyweds in my family cling to one another and "look towards the hills", although the pandemic forced one to seek unemployment not even a month after exchanging vows. I witnessed another relative marry his fiancée, in spite of the pandemic. During the reception, he stood before us all and thanked us by saying, "It wouldn't have been a wedding, without each of you."

My family also buried a twenty-three-year-old due to the pandemic. Words cannot express my sorrow from attending that funeral. Although these twenty-year-olds may not have been considered "babes" due to their ages, their words, actions, and legacies have encouraged me and caused me to give GOD all the praise! Thank you, Jesus, for the young people in my life! I encourage you to listen, support, lead by example, and inspire a young person in YOUR life.

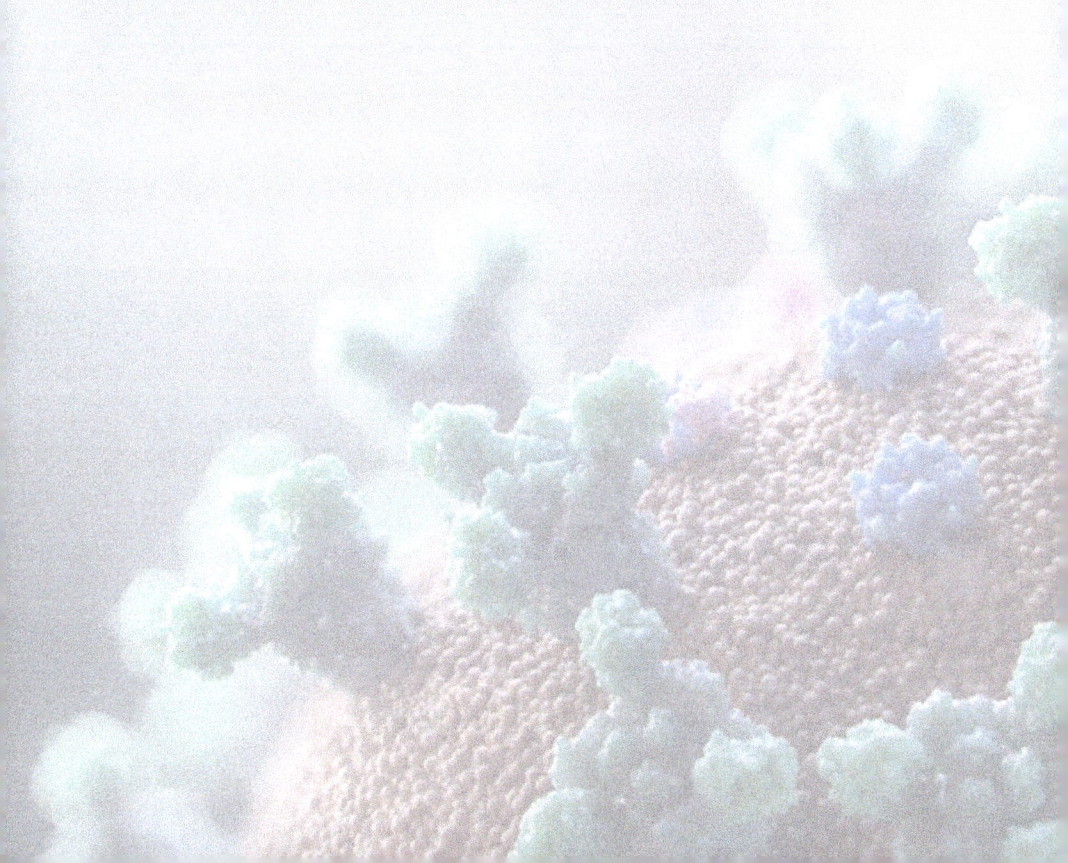

This concludes *Confinement Chronicles, Volume VII – Out of the Mouths of Our Babes* – as inspired by Matthew 21:16 which states:

Do you hear what these children are saying?" they asked him.
"Yes," replied Jesus, "have you never read,
"'From the lips of children and infants
you, Lord, have called forth your praise[a]?"

As read in the New International Version of the Bible

There were more children that had something to share ... something to say ... something to scream about. If you know a child that has been affected by this pandemic, and you believe their story will help another, send an email to AspecialAnnouncement@gmail.com These stories shall continue!

I want to leave you with our foundational scripture for this volume. It comes to us from the book of Matthew, Chapter 21, beginning with verse 14 and ending with verse 17. It reads:

Then the blind and the lame came to Him in the temple, and He healed them. [15] *But when the chief priests and scribes saw the wonderful things that He did, and the children crying out in the temple and saying, "Hosanna to the Son of David!" they were [c]indignant* [16] *and said to Him, "Do You hear what these are saying?"*

And Jesus said to them, "Yes. Have you never read,
'Out of the mouth of babes and nursing infants You have perfected praise'?"
[17] *Then He left them and went out of the city to Bethany, and He lodged there.*

Watch the babes in your life. They have perfected praise!

Be safe and BEE Blessed

Sincerely,
Evangelist Angie BEE

VOLUME VIII

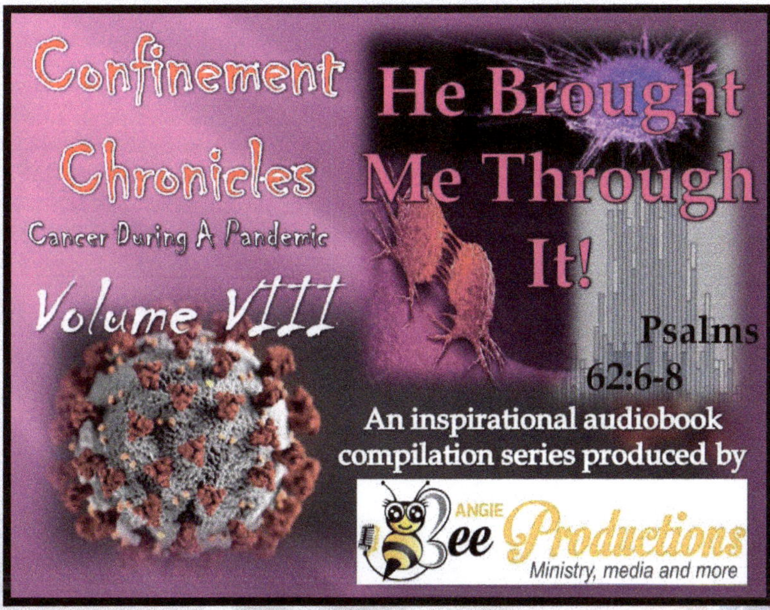
Confinement
Chronicles
Cancer During A Pandemic
Volume VIII
He Brought Me Through It!
Psalms 62:6-8
An inspirational audiobook compilation series produced by
ANGIE Bee Productions
Ministry, media and more

T*rust in him at all times, you people; pour out your hearts to him, for God is our refuge.* Psalm 62:8 New International Version of the Bible.

This scripture SCREAMED out to me this year, as several physicians mentioned the "possibility" of cancer in my body as I sat in their offices. I spent months in pain, weeks medicated, and even more time in recovery from a surgical procedure that eventually found Adenomyosis, *Vasculitis AND Angitiis*. Based upon the symptoms that I began exhibiting in November 2019, the doctor suspected cancer. After enduring a hysterectomy in the midst of a pandemic on June 25, 2020, there was NO CANCER FOUND!

I continued to rejoice when I opened a letter dated August 17, 2020, and read the words:

"We are pleased to tell you that your imaging study shows no significant abnormalities."

Just the sound of the word "cancer" can send chills through your mind and soul. They tell us that "Faith Without Works is Dead." Well, I have heard stories from people that did the work, and their faith grew stronger. I know of others that chose the faith ***without*** the works, and they left others behind in this world with an improved faith in God. Cancer can do that to you. I have seen it happen in other families, and I have lived through it in my own family.

Both my grandmother and HER mother were breast cancer survivors (on my mother's side of the family). While growing up, I was blessed to be the eldest child of the fifth generation on BOTH sides of my family! My maternal grandmother "Gram Gram" was born in 1927, and her mother "BigMama" was born in either 1909 or 1910. Throughout my life, there was always a conversation as to what year she was born. She always said that she was born in 1909, yet my mother found her as an infant listed on the 1910 census. I do know that she lived until the Twin Towers were hit on 9/11. As she lay in the hospital waiting for me to arrive, all of the flights were grounded, so I had to load my

CONFINEMENT CHRONICLES | 161

family up in my car to drive from Orlando to Detroit. Our car made it as far as Atlanta ... but that's a story for another time.

I was in college when my mother told me that my great-grandmother had breast cancer. "Call your Bigmama," she said. It was Sunday, so the long-distance phone rates on the "home phone" were really low (we didn't have cell phones in the early 1980s). My calling-card had about thirty minutes on it, so I wanted to spend that time talking to Bigmama.

"Hey, Bigmama, it's Angie! How you doing?" I asked her.

"Not too good, baby. The doctor wanna cut on me," was her response.

"Why do they wanna cut on you?" I asked, pretending not to know what was wrong.

"You know what they always find in us women. They found it in me, and now they wanna cut it off," she aggressively stated. There was pain in her voice, along with an "I'm not playing with you today, Angie" kind of firmness. I didn't know how to respond. It was the fall of 1983, and I was a freshman on the campus of Wilberforce University, on a full academic scholarship. I had homework to complete before Monday morning classes; I still had to call my boyfriend on what was left of this thirty-minute calling card; and I didn't know how to respond.

"When you coming to see me?" she asked. "I got some slips, stockings, and panties for you from JCPenney's," she added.

And that was how she told me ... make a statement, and then show me some love through undergarments, purchased on the only credit card she had.

A few weeks later, my mom called to tell me that my grandmother (her mother and Bigmama's only child) was also diagnosed with breast cancer. When my grandmother realized that her mother had cancer, she went and got herself checked out. I have also heard stories that my grandfather actually found the lump in GramGram's breast, but if they told me that story, they would also have to admit that granddaddy was TOUCHING her breast, so ... LOL!

The bottom line is that both mother and daughter lost a breast to cancer within a span of a few months. My grandmother was forced to go on disability after her surgery because of the aggressive nature of the procedure; they took so much muscle from under her arm that she could barely lift it over her head. My grandmother had been a "Visiting Nurse" before her diagnosis, so she was no longer able to care for others after "they butchered her" as she referred to it. Neither of them expected to survive after surgery because they believed that "once they open-you-up and the air hits that cancer, it spreads and you die." My mother's faith in God was strong enough to hold them both. Not only did they survive the after-treatments, but each of them lived into their 90s, just as feisty as ever!

Due to this medical history on the maternal side of my family, I was able to start receiving my annual mammogram at the age of thirty. A couple of years ago, they thought they found something, and I endured another exam. Praise God, that test came back negative. Then, I heard the word "cancer" coming out of my doctor's mouth in the fall of 2019. You will hear more about THAT later in this audiobook.

During the pandemic, I read stories and heard from people who were diagnosed with cancer, and paying tributes to others who they had lost to cancer. Each of them gave God praise for what they witnessed during that trial. We are prepared to share these stories with you, through this, Volume VIII "He Brought Me Thorough It!" of *Confinement Chronicles*.

We have had several volumes of *Confinement Chronicles* from faith to Alopecia Awareness. After the devastating and emotional loss of both "The Black Panther" and "RBG" to cancer, we have produced this volume to spread cancer awareness and offer hope. In one-way-or-another, these inspirational audiobooks will continue to encourage us to hear the Word of God, encourage us to write, and encourage us to share.

This is Volume VIII, and although it may have been delivered to listeners a bit out of order (Volume IX debuted on September 15, 2020), these words that you are about to experience are WELL WORTH THE WAIT!

And now, for our first contribution...

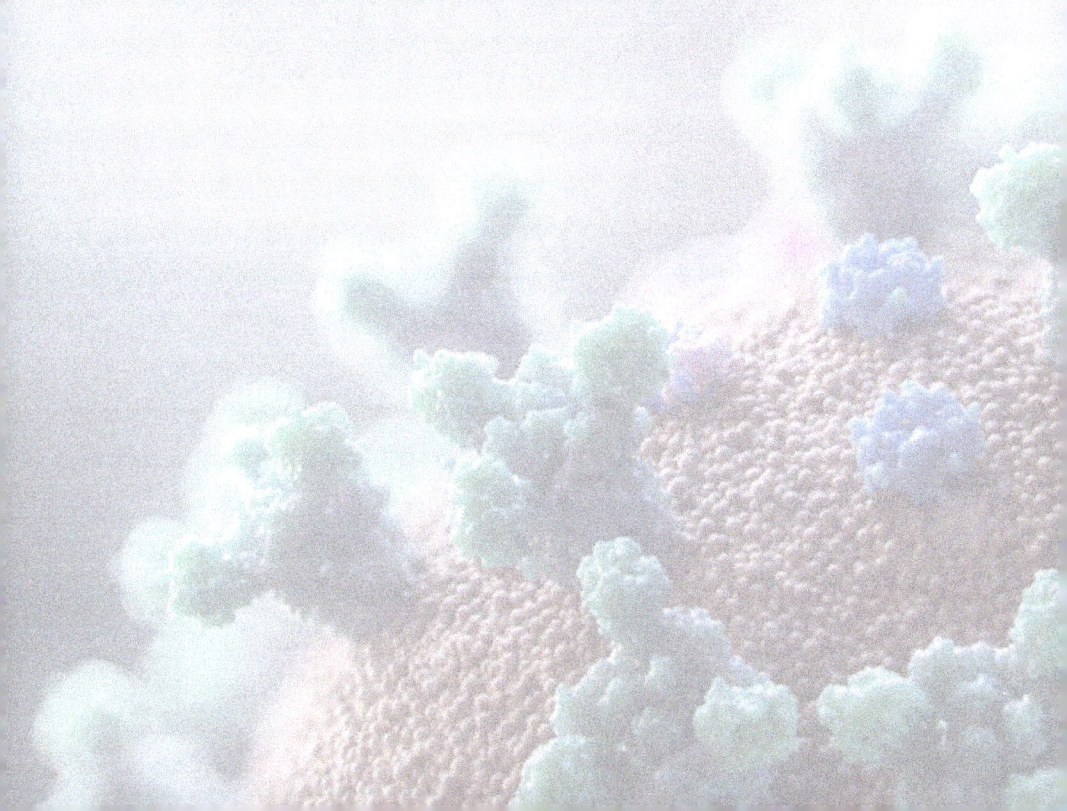

SEEDS OF DOUBT

Angie Cowan

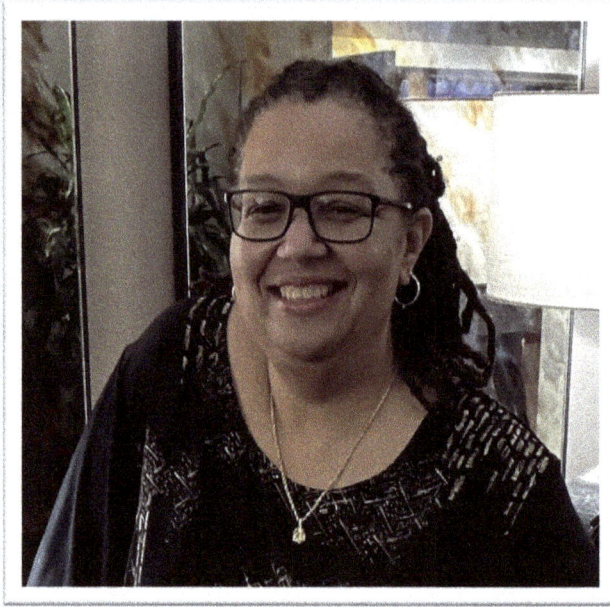

W hen I was first approached about writing this piece, I was excited, but then I allowed a seed of doubt to enter my mind. *Why me? I am not a writer so why would anyone want to hear anything from me?* The doubt took a real grip on me and prevented me from doing anything. A message was given at church that reminded me to keep going, persevere through the doubt, and tell my story. Don't get tripped up again. Truth be told, in that message I was reminded that lately I had been allowing any wall I hit, a "no," or a distraction stop me from moving forward. In that moment, I had to repent and pray to God to help me. In that moment, I remembered the awful day I was diagnosed with MS, and I wondered, "Why me?"

A few years later, I was diagnosed with cancer, and again I wondered, "Why me?" To be honest after dealing with MS, I had automatically eliminated myself from getting cancer. It's funny because Isaiah 55:8-9 says, *"For my thoughts are not your thoughts, neither are your ways my ways,' declares the LORD. "As the heavens are higher than the earth, so are my ways higher than your ways and my thoughts than your thoughts."*

It was the year I was diagnosed with stage 3 colon cancer that I fasted for the first time in my life. It surprised me that my spirit was at peace with doing it that year because, in years before, I never gave thought to fasting, and giving up meat was equivalent to asking me to pull a tooth out of my mouth. However, I persevered and on the last part of the fast, I truly understood the meaning of Philippians 4:13, *I can do all things through Christ who strengthens me.* It was what I learned in that scripture that turned my "why me" of the cancer diagnosis to, *Well, it's here, and now I have to deal with it. So, what am I going to do about it? Trust God and get through it.*

While I didn't understand it then, I would eventually come to understand Jeremiah 29:11, *"For I know the plans I have for you," declares the LORD, "plans to prosper you and not to harm you, plans to give you hope and a future."* It's that statement that let me know "why me." At the early stages of this journey, I said I'm far too young to deal with this. Again, it wasn't going away just because I thought I was too young. The first leg of the journey was surgery. I was told the day after learning of the cancer that I needed to have surgery right away. In years past, about this time, I would've gone into this "why me, woe is me" depression. I soon learned that with God all things are possible. That weekend, I heard a lady repeat what the pastor told her when she received a cancer diagnosis. *Don't claim what's not yours so you don't have cancer, you have a diagnosis.* That one statement stuck in my mind and kept me from sulking. The surgery was a colectomy or a colon resection. All the love and prayers I received before, during, and after the surgery from family and friends gave me the life support I needed to push through post-surgery, to get out of the hospital, and move forward. I was told to prepare for a five-to-seven-day hospital stay. When I told the doctor I was determined to get out sooner rather than later, she said, "I like your enthusiasm, but because of the surgery you're having, prepare to stay the entire time." Here was my first challenge. The surgery was on a Wednesday morning. The following Monday, five days later, I was home. After getting home and trying to rest, I received a call with the next blow—a devastating blow. The doctor called to say that while the surgery went well, and she was able to remove everything, the test results came back from the tissue they removed – it was stage 3 cancer. Only two of the seven polyps removed tested positive; however, the cancer showed up in my lymph nodes which meant I had to undergo chemotherapy. I hung up the phone, and right then and right there declared that once I completed chemotherapy, I would be cured of cancer and MS.

Now, I was on to part two of my cancer journey. By this time, I felt like I had seen more doctors in that short time than I had seen in my entire life. Now, I was off to see more doctors. First, back to surgery to have a port placed in my chest and to the oncologist who would monitor me during the chemo treatment. By the grace of God, he had an awesome ARNP (Advanced Registered Nurse Practitioner). She broke down everything to me -- the drugs they prescribed and what I should expect to happen to me during the treatment.

I got a call from a home health agency that was also part of the treating team. For the next six months, every other week my routine was going to the hospital to get a blood test and start the treatment. When that was over, I would go home where a nurse would come to connect a portable chemo bag to me that I would carry with me for the next two days. On the third day, the nurse would come back to remove the bag and clean the area. After the first treatment, I said "I got this," or so I thought. Almost immediately, the chemo began to affect me physically. I had planned to attend my church's New Year's Eve service ... that was not happening. It was a little scary because I didn't know if this would be just the start of things getting worse. I continued to press on and even decided to go back to work after the two months I was required to stay at home to recover from the surgery. I was advised to stay home and not work, but I was determined to not let this take over my life. So, I would be off from work every other week for chemo treatment day but would carry my portable IV machines with me to work, and the nurse would come to the job to remove the machine from me. I kept on but it certainly was a journey. Although I was working, I had to push my way through the various side effects. Some days were good, and some were not so good. Because I went through this every other week, I felt like every time I started to feel good again, it was time to be knocked down again.

I was attempting to live my life like normal while trying to ignore how I was really feeling. I recall going to an event one evening, and it began to rain. It was just a sprinkle, and no one knew it, but the raindrops that were hitting my arms made me truly miserable, but I kept going – determined not to let this defeat me. The rain finally cleared up and allowed me to enjoy the evening again.

I was also dealing with fatigue. It had become so bad that on some days, I was so exhausted, I had just enough energy to get from the car to my bed. Once I got in the bed, I wouldn't move until the next morning. By this time, I was just about halfway through the treatments and coming up on my next appointment. I woke up that morning and said I didn't want to go anymore. I don't like saying I had given up, but honestly, my body was so tired of getting beaten up, my mind was saying, *Ok, we're over this.*

I told my aunt that I didn't want to do anymore chemo. She told me, "Don't give up now; you're halfway there." She prayed for me and said, "Go ahead, everything is going to be okay." All the way to the hospital, my mind was still in this place where I didn't want to go, but I continued to press my way there. Let me tell you, God certainly knows how to give you what you need, exactly when you need it.

On the very morning I wanted to give up, I arrived for my appointment and started the treatment. One of the cancer-center volunteers that came that day offered to do a paint project. She normally came on a different day, but God moved on her heart to change days. That project was just what I needed to help me get through the rest of the treatments. Every other Monday, she and I worked on this watercolor painting until it was done on my last treatment day. That project kept me from feeling my body braiding down during the hours I was getting these drugs pumped into my system. On the last day of treatment, once you're done, all the available medical staff join you to celebrate the end of the journey. I wanted to ring that bell off the wall because I was so glad to be done.

The third part of the journey was follow-up appointments and tests. Early on in the follow-ups, I worried about recurrence and the cancer coming back. A friend said to me, "If you're gonna trust God, trust God." So, I continued to trust God. Because of a previous MS diagnosis, I had to test for that, too, because I hadn't been receiving any treatments for that at all since the cancer diagnosis. I had an MRI, and the results were really good.

The nurse said to me, "I don't see any movement from the lesions, and the MS seems dormant."

While she wouldn't say I was cured, she said, "If I were you, I wouldn't jump on any new medication right now because you're doing well without it."

In my mind, that was the healing I called right before the chemo treatments got started. Fast forward to now, 2020, a year like nothing we've ever experienced. In the midst of the craziness, God is still blessing. It's been five years since I had my last chemo treatment and officially have been released from the oncologist's care. I am now five years cancer free. I don't take any medication for any illness.

Most people would be surprised if I told them everything that I've been through. Today, I again declare that God has healed me from cancer and MS! The recent passing of Chadwick Boseman affected me a little differently than most. Most people were upset about the loss of the man that brought us *The Black Panther* and the other characters he portrayed, and losing him at such a young age made it even more tragic. It affected me for those reasons, too, but more so because, like him, I was diagnosed with stage 3 colon cancer at a young age – forty-four. This brings me to my final "why me" and why some people are spared, and others aren't.

Seeds of doubt were trying to bottle up everything that I went through when God wanted me to share how he healed me and the things he did along the way to get me from then to now. Last year, I celebrated my 50th birthday. It was a truly awesome birthday. Had I given up, I would not have been alive to celebrate that birthday or to celebrate the life God blessed me to have. So now, I'm here to tell you to keep on running, and keep persevering, no matter what. There's life and blessings and healing on the other side.

BREAST CANCER SURVIVOR

Sharlyne Rogers

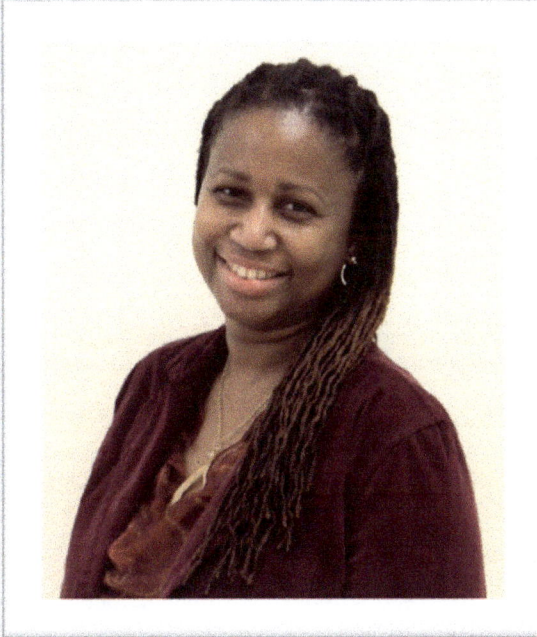

My mother Constance turned eighty-four years young on February 19, 2020, after being diagnosed with, treated for, and eventually healed from breast cancer in her early 70s. She lost both breasts in her brave battle, but not her life. She lost her hair during chemotherapy, but it later grew back healthier than before. She lost her physical strength during the subsequent radiation treatments, but she is still as feisty as ever. She even lost her sense of taste, but I'm quite sure it's back now since she frequently eats ice cream with her lunch.

The day that my mom told me she had breast cancer is foggy but not forgotten. I live in Florida, but she still lives in my home state of California, so this tough conversation had to be done over the phone. She simply said, "I have cancer." I cried because she was crying, and that was a sound that I hadn't heard from her in over three decades. I don't think we were on the phone too long but as soon as we hung up, my tears were quickly dried when I heard the Lord whisper this scripture in my spirit:

This sickness is not unto death, but for the glory of God ... (John 11:4b)

I can't tell you the exact day, month, or year that my mother was diagnosed with cancer, but I do have photo proof that I completed my very first 5K breast cancer walk on October 23, 2010, for the American Cancer Society "Making Strides Against Breast Cancer" event in Orlando. I was selling Avon at the time, so I had a cute and colorful shirt made that had these words on the back: "daughter of Constance Blount - breast cancer SURVIVOR!" I also added that scripture from the book of John, which is what kept my faith going during my mother's recovery. And I always use that prophetic Word to encourage other friends who have battled cancer or had family members who have.

The October breast cancer walk in Downtown Orlando has been a tradition for me for the past 10 years; and although 2020 will be different due to the COVID-19 pandemic, the spirit of healing and fellowship will not be abandoned. I would usually bring my daughter and grandchildren to meet up with a few friends at Lake Eola Park to pray and praise throughout the entire three-mile route. This year, I'll have to take a much less-crowded circle around my own block to promote breast cancer awareness; however, I will still have a team representing my 501c3 nonprofit, Sword of the Spirit Ministries, and accepting donations to help support this important cause. I pray that by next year, we'll be out of confinement!

THIS IS THE STORY ABOUT MY GRANDDADDY KERVOICER

Evangelist Angie BEE

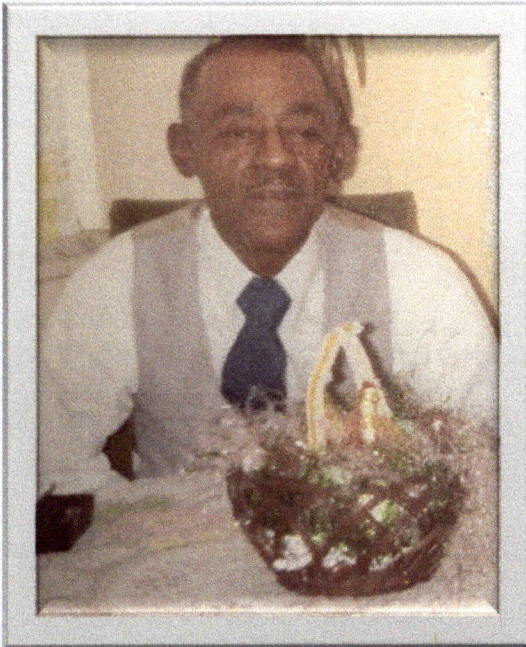

Kervoicer Henderson
May 8th 1925 – July 8, 1989

I had a brief conversation with my sisters for this next segment. I wanted to truly capture how cancer had affected our family, and I wanted to include their memories of our grandfather.

My sister Sonya said, "The most significant thing that I can remember about granddaddy was that he kept complaining that his back was hurting. I remember that he bought a new mattress for his bed, to help him sleep better. We kept bugging him to go to the doctor, and when he finally did, he was dead about a month later. Lung cancer took our beloved granddaddy from us."

My mother said that she accompanied granddaddy to one of his doctor appointments. It was during that visit that they interviewed him to try and better understand the correlation between smoking and lung disease. My mother was shocked when her father replied to the physician's questions by saying, "I started smoking when I was about eight or nine years old. That was the only entertainment that a poor nigga in Macon, Georgia could have, back then."

My sister Tanya added, "I guess he realized around Easter / April / sometime in 1989 that he was sick. I remember that we had a 4th of July gathering, and we wanted him to eat. He pretended to eat but just didn't have an appetite, so we took him outside to lay on the lounge chair to try to get some sun. We were all outside and he said to us:

**'Cancer is not something I would wish on my worst enemy.
It is so painful!'**

He started taking chemo and it forced him to lose a lot of weight in a short amount of time. I think he may have known before, but just didn't tell anybody. He just thought that his back was hurting."

He just wanted to try and stay strong. Tanya says that she was with him the day before he passed so Gram Gram could run to the store. She said, "He was trying to communicate something that he needed, but his voice was gone, and he couldn't get it out."

He passed on a Saturday. I remember because I was at the church volunteering to fold the Sunday morning programs. My sister Sonya and my dad came up to the church to pick me up and tell me that Granddaddy was in the hospital on a ventilator. He was lying in the hospital bed with Gram Gram sitting next to him. She was reciting the Lord's Prayer; it was really hard for her to say goodbye to her husband. Granddaddy's eyes were wide open while they puffed those drugs into him to try to keep him alive. I remember the ventilator and all of that. I was probably about nineteen years old.

Tanya went on to say, "Mom was looking out the window from the hospital cafeteria, and she saw a vision of a well-dressed man looking at her through the window and waving good-bye to her. It had been hard for her to see him wasting away like that. In that moment, our mother knew that her father was gone."

Tanya concluded by saying that our dad said that (well before the diagnosis), "Granddaddy was outside painting the house railings and making sure the house looked wonderful. He was always good at that. I guess he just wanted to be sure that everything was perfect."

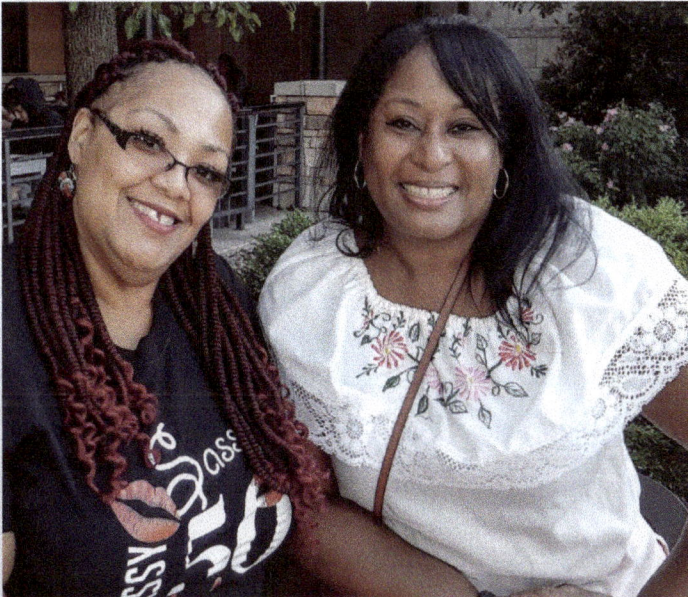

Thank you to my sisters Sonya & Tanya Bennett for their contributions to this dedication!

This next story is my personal testimony. You may read it and the empowering story of others in the upcoming book entitled, *Daily Dose of Declarations*, a collaborative project, written by Melanie Bonita, and including the following story written by me, Evangelist Angie BEE.

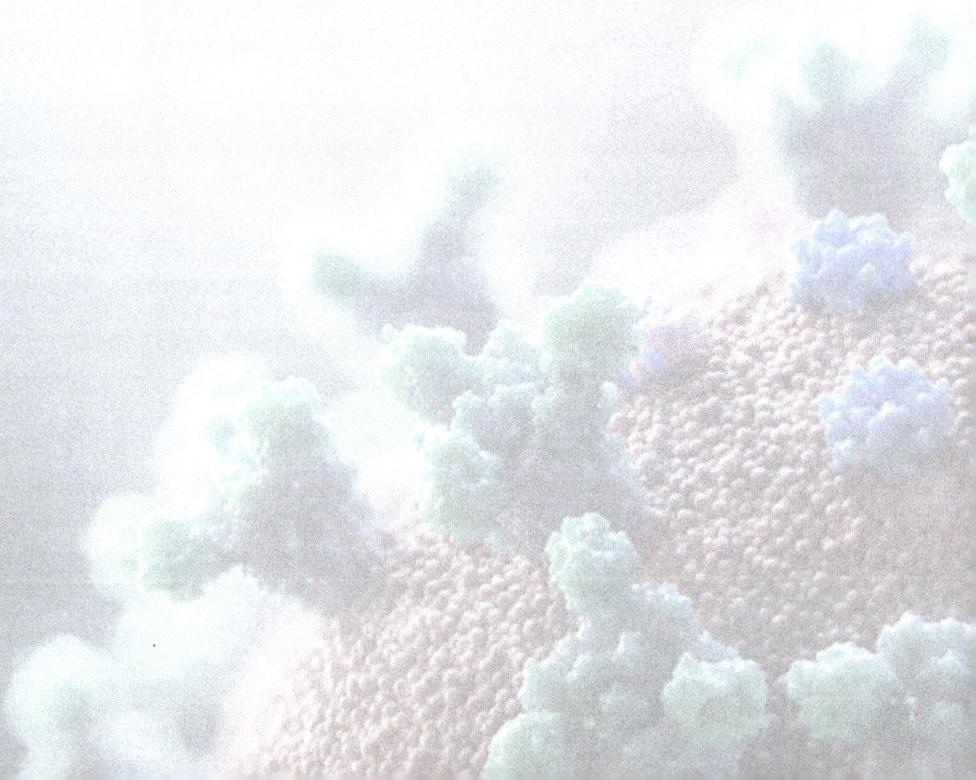

THE HYSTERECTOMY DECLARATION: NOTHING COMPARES TO GOD

(As inspired by the song "Nothing Compares 2 U" by Prince)

Evangelist Angie BEE

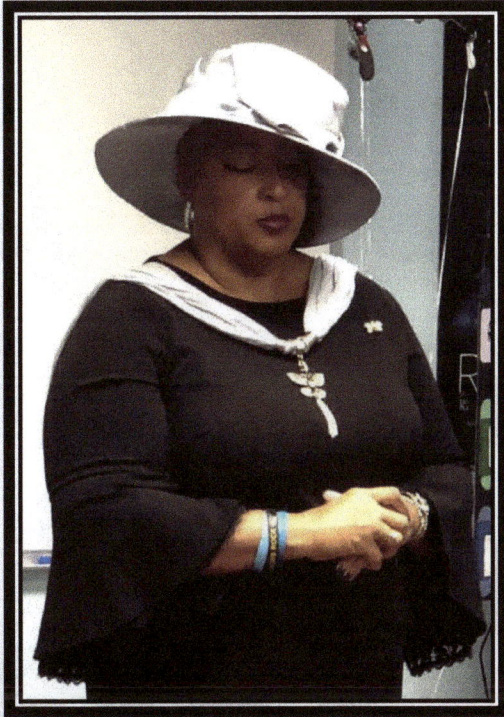

It's been 7 hours and 14 days, since you took my womb away.
Oh Lord, I need you.

I don't leave my home and I sleep all day.
Oh God, I feel you!

Since it's been gone I can feel my body changing...
The constant pain is just a bad dream.

I wait for the doctor to call me;
I look forward to the news that I am cancer-free! But here's a clue...
Nothing compares to the comfort I get from God.

As the days progress without my womb,
I'll share my story with all who care to hear;
And pray that it will lead others to Christ!

3 John 2
*Dear friend, I pray that you may enjoy good health and that all may go well
with you, even as your soul is getting along well.*

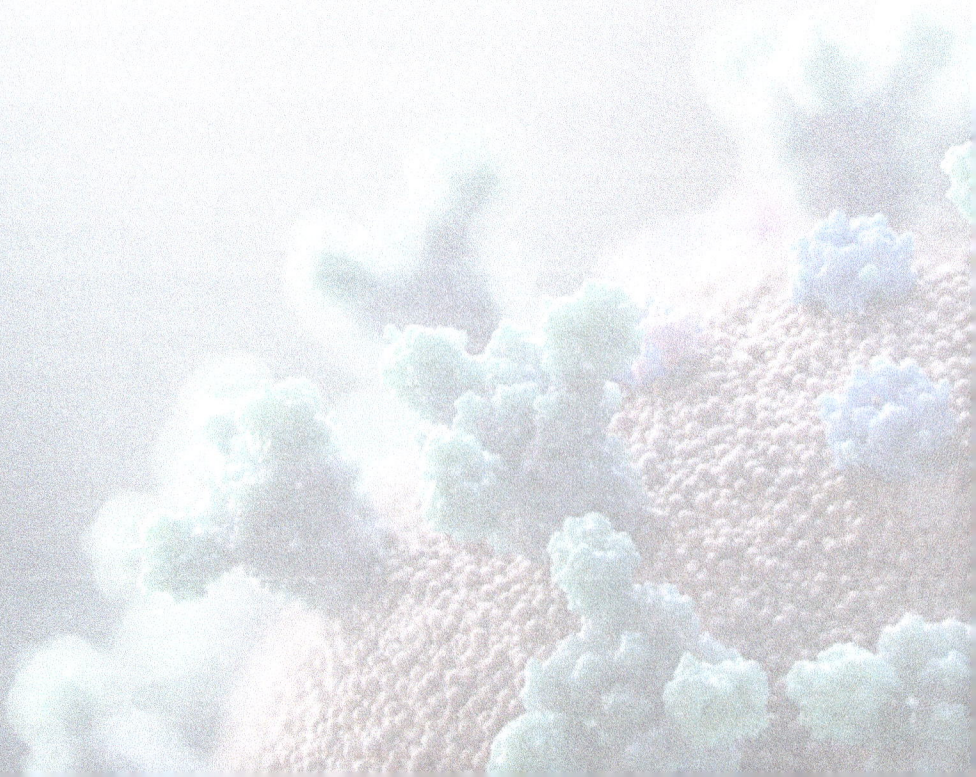

MY MOMMA - HATTIE NEAL

May 20, 1926 - October 19, 1964

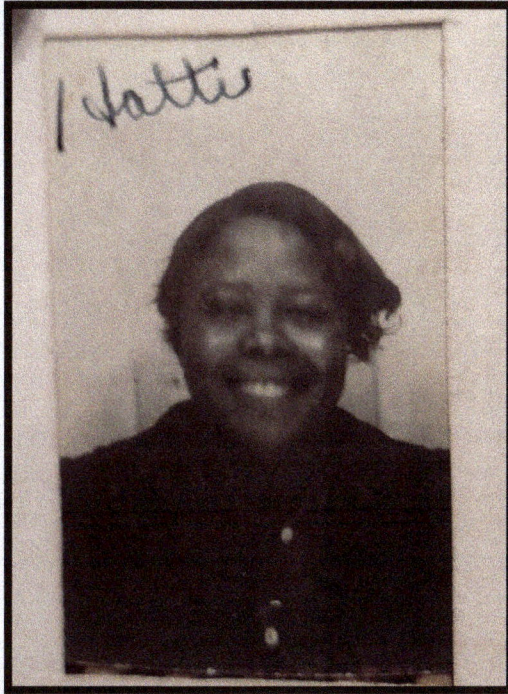

A Dedication of Love

From Bartee

My mom loved to play the piano. We had one of those old pianos with the scrolling sheet music in it. She smoked Pall Mall cigarettes, and she liked Wild Irish Rose! I don't remember a lot about my mother except that she loved her kids. Her death certificate hangs on my wall that reflects her date of death as October 19, 1964, as the result of

Pneumonia due to Metastatic Breast Carcinoma

May she rest in peace, and "I will see you, when I get there, Momma."

Love, Your Son

Bartee keeps a laminated souvenir obituary from the funeral home. I will now read it as a reflection of her bio.

Services for Mrs. Hattie Neal of 1319 8th Avenue took place on a Saturday at 11 AM in the Good Hope Baptist Church, which she was a member. Mrs. Neal, who died Monday in Akron City Hospital, was a native of Monticello, Florida, and a resident of Akron and Barberton for 30 years. She leaves three sons, Wilbert Lawrence Bartee, Eddie and Eugene Neal and a daughter Brenda Bartee, all of Akron; a brother and five sisters in Florida and New York.

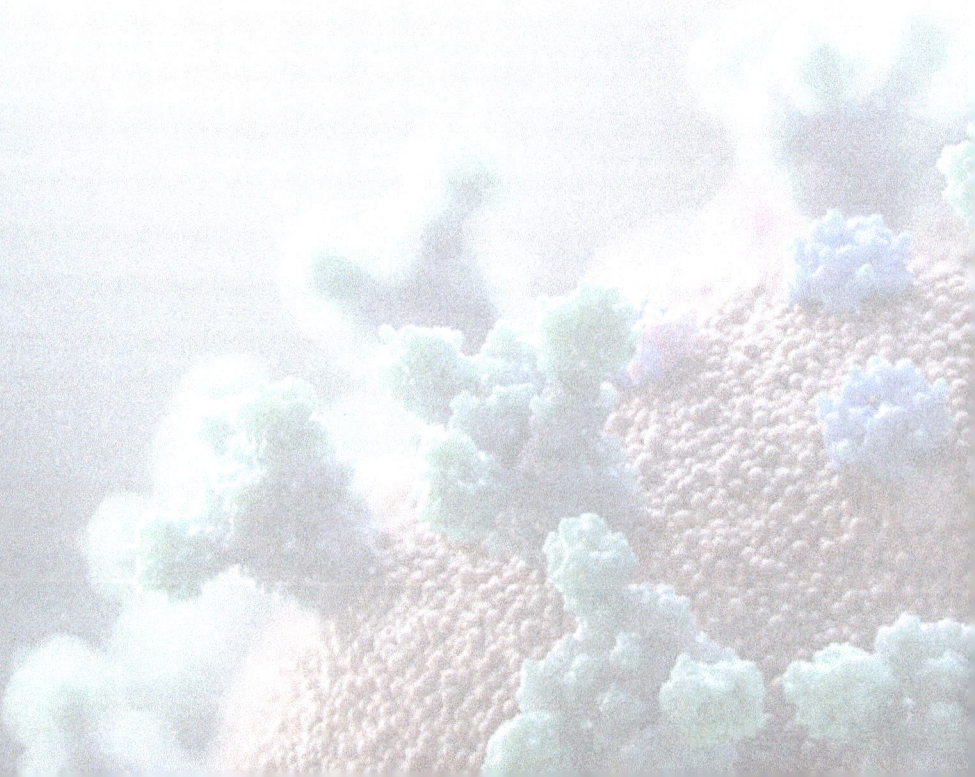

Thomara La Toye Latimer

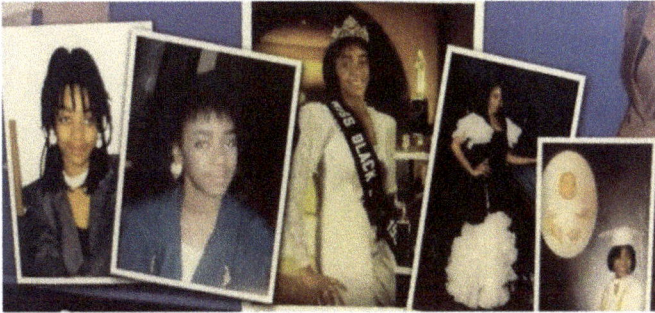

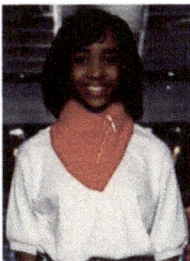

Thomara LaToye Latimer

Miss Perfect Teen Pageant

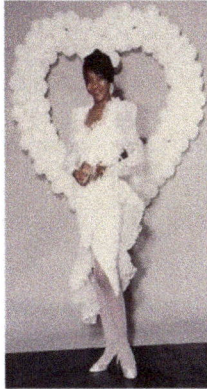

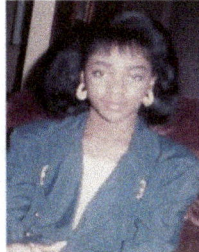

Entry for Miss Teen U.S.A

'Helping Families Face the Challenges of Cancer'

February 19, 1975 - December 10, 1997

Cancer places men, women, boys, and girls in an *"elite club"* that they would "never voluntarily" join. Thomara became a member of that *"elite club"* at the beginning of her senior year at Grand Valley State University in 1996.

Thomara was an extremely precocious child entering kindergarten at four years old. She truly loved the arts. At five, she began dancing with performing and competition groups at Northwest School of Dance. She also sang in the church choir and began learning piano and violin. During her second-grade year at

Presentation, Our Lady of Victory School, she was asked to join the school's cheerleading squad that was made up of girls in grades six, seven, and eight. These girls not only cheered at school events like basketball games, they also performed at local competitions.

Middle school advanced her talents as well as her interest in pageants. When Thom entered high school, she asked to enter those pageants. Her first pageant was Miss Perfect Teen. She did not win but set specific goals for the next pageant. Her next pageant was Miss Teen U.S.A. Again, she did not win. But her dynamic belief in God never permitted her to give up. With this belief and determination, she entered the Miss Black Star of Detroit Pageant and won based on swimsuit, eveningwear, and her performance of the violin. She was told that playing her violin was a poor choice for performance, but the judges and audience gave her a standing ovation.

Thom enjoyed learning. The excellence she achieved in school *earned* her induction into the high school's *Scholar's Plus Program* and the *National Honor Society*. She enjoyed four years of Spanish and the Spanish Club, four years on the student council board, three years on the volleyball team, and being voted MVP by the Southeastern Michigan Association.

In 1992, Thomara matriculated to Grand Valley State University in Allendale, Michigan, on a full scholarship in the field of biomedical science. Her passion since junior high school was to become a pediatrician. She adored little children after baby-sitting for neighbors and friends during her years in high school. She became a *Big Sister* and worked diligently with children in Grand Rapids, Michigan. The initial *Knowledge Pursuit Program* for children, based at True Love Baptist Church in Detroit, was developed and implemented by Thomara and three other young college freshmen. The next summer, Thomara volunteered to work with children in the Grand Rapids *Summer Journeys Program*. This program was also designed to mentor and keep children off the street while developing their talents and skills.

Thom (Thomas) + ara (Barbara) Thomara was diagnosed with cancer at the age
of 21, November 4, 1996. After a valiant fight, she lost the battle on December 10,
1997.

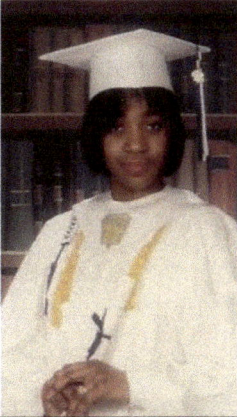

National Honor Society

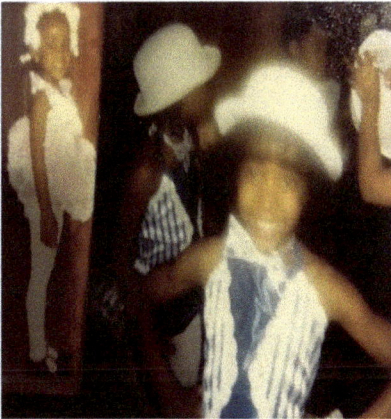

Thomara dancing with the Minilites
Performing Troup

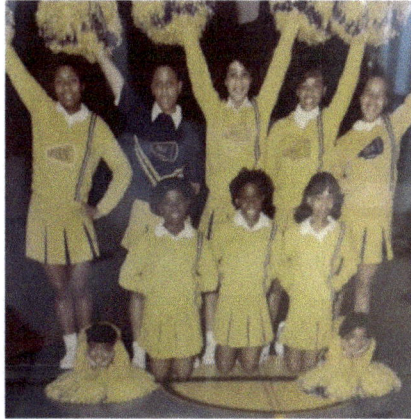

Thomara, bottom left holding chin, with her
cheering squad

The History of the Thomara Latimer Cancer Foundation
A Legacy of Love, Help, & Hope

Life changes when cancer appears. Thomara, at twenty-one, was a senior at
Grand Valley State University, preparing for her passion to become a
pediatrician when her change took place. Although she transitioned on

December 10, 1997, her legacy of life and helping others continues through the Thomara Latimer Cancer Foundation.

The Thomara Latimer Foundation was established on July 14, 1998. Family, friends, physicians, nurses, and clergy came together at the home of Thomas & Barbara Latimer to honor the memory of one who touched their lives in so many special ways. This group pledged to dedicate themselves to serving the needs of others. Thus, a 501(C)(3) charitable organization was formed to provide compassionate, valuable services and resources to pediatric and young adult cancer patients and provide scholarships to students in pursuit of any area of medical studies. More specifically, the foundation's goals were the following:

- To provide funds for cancer treatment or medication not covered by insurance,
- To provide funds for homecare assistance, including food and gas cards,
- To provide transportation to and from treatment, physician and/or support facilities,
- To provide special needs funds for wigs/head coverings for diagnosis or treatment related hair loss or prostheses,
- To provide respite to families and/or caregivers,
- To assist with final arrangements for families without life insurance, AND
- Provide scholarships to students in pursuit of any area of medicine.

Needing seed money to begin, the board of directors and the membership planned two activities: a raffle and the First Annual Scholarship Gala. The keynote speaker for the first event was Thomara's oncologist, Dr. Roman Franklin. Other keynote speakers include the Honorable Former Mayor of Benton Harbor, Emma J. Hull; Donald Williams, Dean of Students Affairs-Grand Valley State University; Dr. Verdie Robinson, Dean of Christian Education-Science Teacher; Dr. Al Calvert, author and radio talk-show host; former Chief of Police, City of Detroit; Ella Bully-Cummings, Chief of Police, City of Detroit; Benny Napoleon; Lonny Joe, M.D.; Rev. Herbert B. Robinson,

Jr., D. Min., Pastor of True Love Missionary Baptist Church; Herman B. Gray, M.D., President of Children's Hospital of Michigan; and Rev. Dr. Charles G. Adams, Pastor of Hartford Memorial Baptist Church.

The format of our program changed in two thousand thirteen-fourteen. Comedienne, Crystal P wowed our supporters. Master/Mistress of Ceremony have included Huel Perkins, Fanchon Stinger, and Anquinette Jamison from Fox 2 News; Rhonda Walker, Channel 4; Carolyn Clifford, Channel 7; City Councilwoman Saunteel Jenkins; Dr. Deborah Smith-Pollard FM 98 WJLB Radio; Roderick Marshall; Swanson's Funeral Homes; Kori Chambers, Local 4 News; the Honorable Judges Shannon Holmes and Demetria Brue; and Ellis Liddell. TLCF is extremely blessed that all of these supporters gave their time and support in-kind. Each gala after the first awarded $1,000.00 scholarships. The second awarded four recipients; the third awarded seven; the fourth gala awarded ten; and the fifth and beyond awarded twelve. Special scholarship awards were funded and presented by two families in memory of their beloved: our beloved chairperson for seven years, Mashonda Griffin, and the beloved parents of our founder, Barbara Latimer, charter members, Rev. Chester & Geraldine Hollman.

The outpouring of love is immeasurable. The foundation membership and its supporters have been beyond kind and generous. When funds are limited, the membership will purchase much needed items for patients and their families. For example, an eight-year-old patient in a family of six asked for heaters during a very bad and snowy winter. TLCF family members purchased heaters from their own personal resources. Members have used their personal vehicles to take patients or family members to the grocery store and purchased food for the patient's household. Each year, toys, bicycles, clothing, blankets, and other items are delivered to hospitals and homes by the TLCF members and supporters. Most of our members and supporters have been with us the entire twenty-plus years.

In August 1999, the first proposal was submitted to Black United Fund of Michigan, Inc. (BUF) who awarded the foundation with more than $10,000.00. Subsequent awards have ranged from $10,000 to $15,000. Letters were mailed to various physicians, hospitals, hospices, etc. to let them know who we were and how we could help. Because of BUF, concerts, plays, make-believe teas, skate-athons, and other fundraisers, TLCF has been able to manifest its objectives as well as expand.

The Thomara Latimer Cancer Foundation (TLCF) targets and embraces children and young adults who are facing the "challenges of cancer." There are many groups and organizations who are walking, running, and racing for a cure, which is vitally, vitally, necessary. But what about the more than 800,000 people who are struggling with this disease daily whose lives go un-served? Through referrals from Karmanos Institute social workers, Children's Hospital, the American Cancer Society, Hospices of Michigan, the Leukemia Foundation of Michigan and personal requests, TLCF has assisted hundreds. Not only were we able to manifest our initial goals, we were also able to expand our homecare to paying mortgages for patients in jeopardy of losing their homes. Utilities are paid in order to keep our cancer patients warm during the winter. Agreements have been established with Rite Aid in Clarkston and others that approved cancer patients, through TLCF, to receive their medication as needed without worrying about financial issues. Transportation was expanded as the need arose for parents who required daily transportation for pediatric cancer patients. It seemed easier to have their cars repaired than scheduling and implementing transportation services.

Thom's Place, established in 2007, provides two programs: Healing Hearts and NutriNaught Healthy Acts. Healing Hearts provides grief counseling to young people who are dealing with the loss of a parent or sibling, and adults who have lost a child or other loved ones. NutriNaught educates young people and their families on nutritional lifestyle changes to "Slay the Dragon" called cancer and prevent other life-threatening diseases. Nutrition is the key to being "one less" victim of cancer! Please visit our website at www.thomlatimercares.org to view the fourteen suggestions toward a healthier life, hopefully cancer free.

Thom's place is a place where pediatric and young adult patients can find friendship, companionship, help, and hope. TLCF will expand its programs, services, and outreach to accommodate young people in the community, schools, churches, and neighborhood organizations. Currently, the downside of

TLCF is that our geographical limitation only permits us to service the state of Michigan.

Volunteers are needed to ensure our mission! The diagnosis of cancer is hard! Finding help should not be.

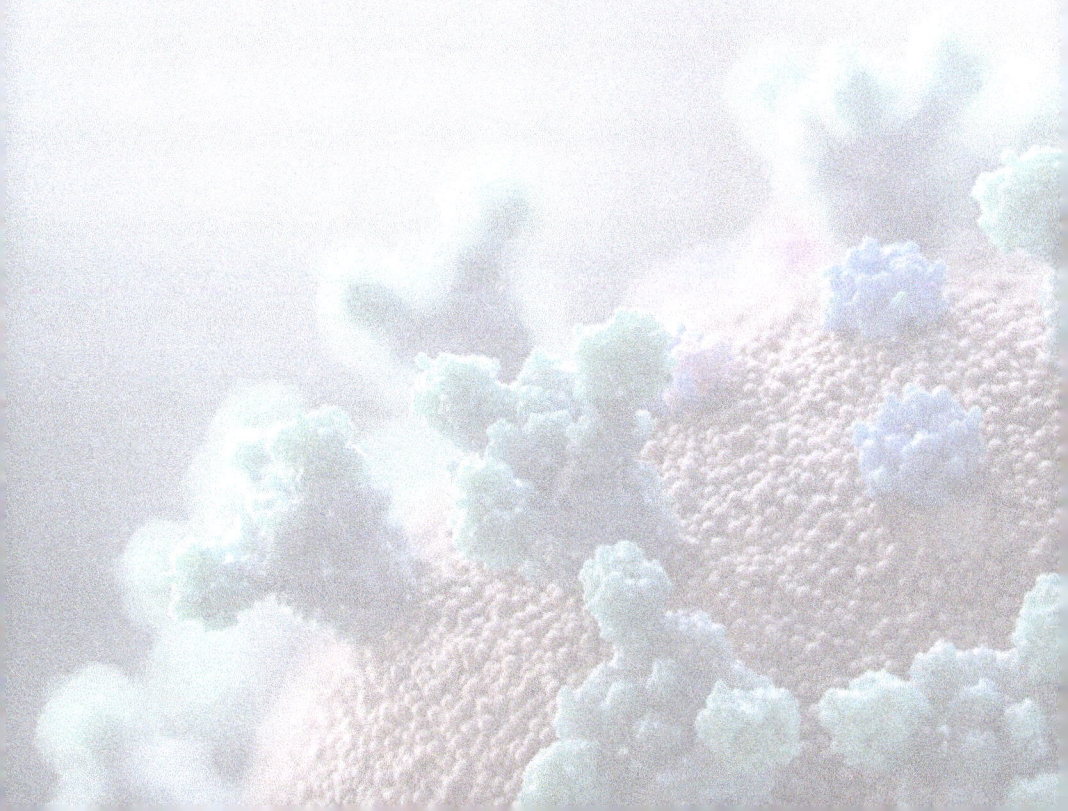

This concludes Confinement Chronicles, Volume VIII.

These stories shall continue!

Be safe and BEE Blessed

Sincerely,

Evangelist Angie BEE

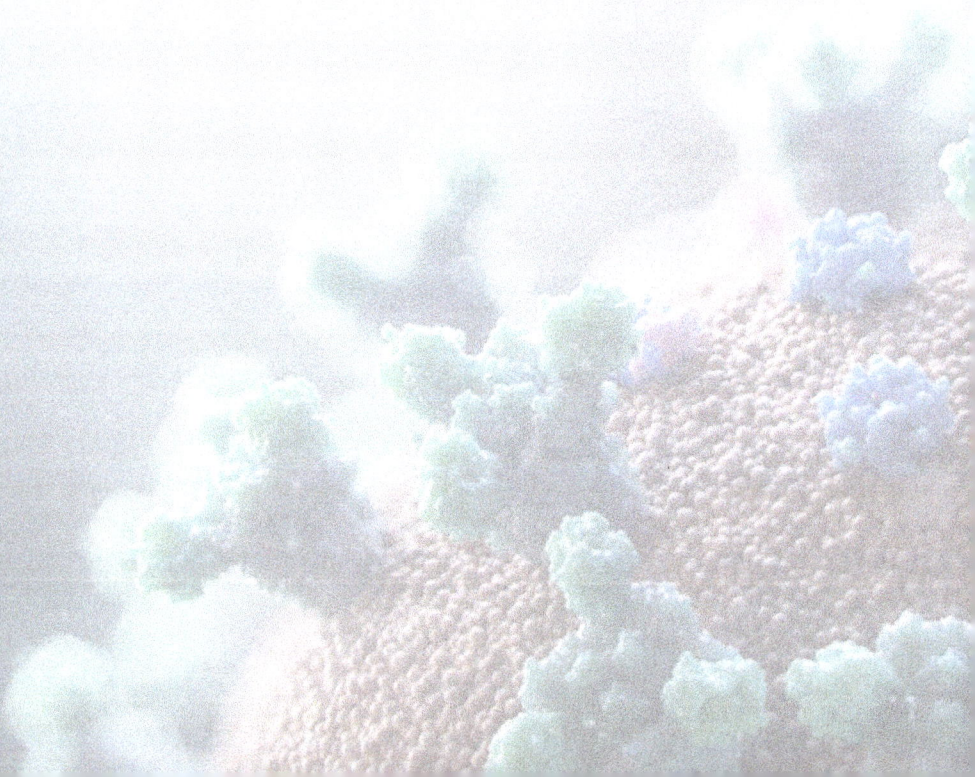

VOLUME IX

Confinement Chronicles

A fundraiser for

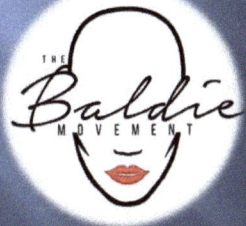

THE Baldie MOVEMENT

Improving our Mental Health by sharing stories of hair loss & survival

#Irefuse to stop being ME!

2 Corinthians 1:3-4

An inspirational audiobook compilation series inspired by the 2020 Pandemic. Produced by

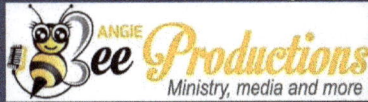

ANGIE Bee Productions
Ministry, media and more

During a recent radio interview, my husband Bartee and I were asked about the Bold Beautiful & Bald Beauty Bazaar. This Alopecia Awareness weekend is an annual fundraiser that takes place in Daytona Beach, Florida, each September, during Alopecia Awareness month. As I shared my hair loss story with the audience, and my husband contributed his thoughts, a beautiful revelation of God's goodness and direction began to unfold before my very eyes. If I had not begun to lose my hair more than twenty years ago, I would not have been able to encourage another person on their journey of hair loss and re-discovery. I am grateful for that revelation!

Now, as we present these stories of hair loss for our Alopecia Awareness audiobook volume, I see how that re-discovery is present in each of our authors. The beginning of our stories may be similar:

- we started losing our hair
- someone noticed and told us that we were losing our hair
- we covered our hair loss in a variety of ways

But now we are each serving a greater calling by helping others in our own special way!

From hair loss to a greater purpose! LOOK AT GOD!

We have arrived at Volume IX and, although it may have been delivered to listeners a bit out of order (Volume VII debuted on September 1, 2020) these words that you are about to experience are WELL WORTH THE WAIT!

And now, for our first contribution...

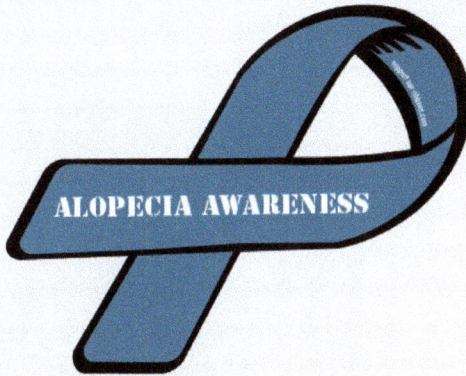

SUMMARY OF MY HAIR STORY

Michelle Walters - Johnson

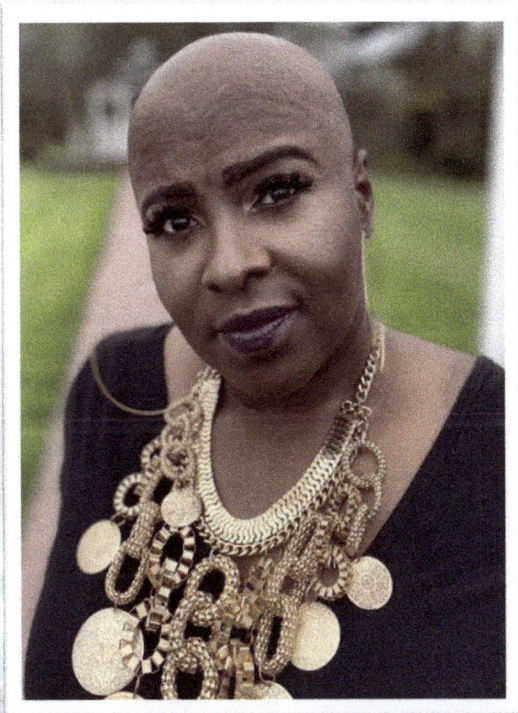

In my experience, my hair loss began at the age of twenty-eight. I was living life, minding my business, and one day my mother came to visit from out of town, and one of her first comments to me was about how thin my hair was. Up until this point, I actually never noticed the hair thinning. But once I really took a look, I came to the realization that my hair was not as thick as it used to be. I have had a love/hate relationship with my hair and with this whole process since then.

My love affair with wigs started after the birth of my daughter fifteen years ago. After her birth, my hair thinned out considerably. I became a professional at learning how to blend my hair with the partial wig. I typically wore them about shoulder length or in a bob so that they were very natural looking. I don't think too many people realized it wasn't my hair. Wigs gave me that extra boost of confidence to try things that I had always wanted to do, but was afraid to, like modeling. But that's a story for another day.

Losing one's hair has a great psychological impact. For many women, hair loss can happen so fast, not giving them enough time to adjust. This can cause some to go into a deep depression. Add to that the fact that they may also be going through medical issues, extreme stress, or some other life impacting drama.

I will never forget the time when I was at a hairdresser appointment with my niece Tiara. We were getting ready to try a treatment, and she prayed over me. That moment is still etched in my head. She prayed that my hair loss would not affect my self-esteem; and I will honestly say from that time forward, I have not psychologically struggled with my hair loss.

Although I have not let Alopecia damage my self-esteem, there are plenty of women that do. This phenomenon gives a new charge to my business, instead of focusing on only creating wigs, I focus on helping women with alopecia feel better about themselves. I have been privileged to influence them to embrace their natural beauty and feel proud about showing their beautiful bald heads; and then if they desire, finding the right wig or wigs that further enhance their natural beauty. By coming forward with my truth, I believe that I have found my profound purpose.

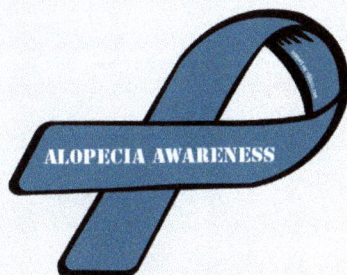

THE ADVENTURES OF A BALDIE....

Lorna Mastin

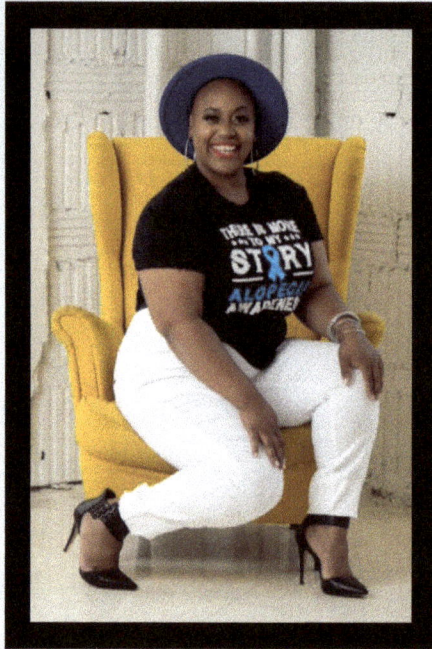

Growing up in Southfield, Michigan, one of my fondest moments was getting my hair done. I had a very nice, soft texture of hair with great length. I was like my mom's personalized Barbie doll. Every hairstyle she wanted to try, she did it on me. I wasn't tender-headed, and I could sit there for hours. Some of my favorite hair styles were latch hook, twisties, and braids. One day, I noticed this tiny little bald spot. When I showed my mom, we thought maybe one of the braids had pulled it out from its tightness. Anywho, we decided to make an appointment for the dermatologist to examine everything, but we honestly didn't think anything of it.

One very cold day on February, the 14th to be exact, in the year of 2002, I went in for my appointment with the dermatologist. I was excited because I was able to get out of school early, but at the same time, attempting to be focused, because we had a volleyball game that day at 4 PM. (I did not play when it came to athletics; I'm very competitive.) So, my mom and I arrived, sat down, and in came the doctor. He examined my head and casually said, "Yeah ... looks like you have Alopecia." I had never heard of it, never knew anyone with it, and could not tell you where it came from. They said it could be hereditary or it could be triggered by stress. I was a little stressed as a teenager, but isn't everybody? So, I thought.

My mom asked about treatment, and it was then that the doctor shared the bitter reality that there was no cure, but we could "try" a few things. (I was thinking, *I know they don't think I'm going to be a guinea pig.*) So, they told us about these cortisone injections that work for some people, and that we could try it. I cried my eyes out asking for another option because I had a game that day, and I didn't think I could handle getting shots in my head and playing. They decided to give me some steroids that I could only take for a month because if I took too many, they could cause kidney failure. So, essentially I had thirty days to prepare my mind for the injections.

When I went back the following Monday, the injections began. Hair would grow in one spot then fall out again. We played this cat and mouse game for four years. Each month I'd go, and I would get anywhere from one hundred to one hundred twenty-six (100-126) injections in my head at a time. OOOoouch! In my senior year of high school, we tried one more thing. I was sent to a specialist, and we tried a light box treatment which ended up looking just like a tanning booth. The idea was that the UV light would stimulate the growth on my head. Well, after a year of that, the end result was actually little to no hair growth, and it tanned the rest of my face. So, my face ended up being darker than the rest of my body. At that point, I had had it! I was over the treatments because nothing was completely successful. Sometimes, I was able to cover up the areas where my hair fell out, and other times I wasn't, and had to wear wigs. Now, these wigs are not what the lace fronts look like today! They were the ones your great-grandmother wore that slid to the right or the left if you turned your head too quickly! An absolute disaster! I remember my ponytail clip falling off while trying to steal second base during a softball game. Or, the time my wig came off while playing volleyball. Or, it sliding alllll the way to the right during a meet as I threw the shot out in disgust! Not to mention all of this happening during high school, where absolutely everything matters. (But not really.)

I managed to make it through high school and decided for all treatments to come to an end. At fourteen, I knew God had a purpose for me experiencing this, but just wasn't sure what it was. Years had gone by, and I still hadn't met anyone with this same condition or that even looked like me and had alopecia. As time progressed, my hair started to grow back. It got really long, too. I was just waiting on my edges to come in. I had gotten married, had a great sew-in, and I thought I was in the clear. Unless you were blood family or really close friends, many still didn't know I suffered from Alopecia, but it didn't bother me as much because I could wear sew-ins to cover it up.

Welp, in 2015, I got pregnant with my son, and of course my hair grew like crazy, but when he came out in 2016, so did ALLLLLLL of my hair. This was tough. I was trying to hold onto the little I did have. I felt bad for my now ex-husband because he liked hair—long hair—and n order to give him that, I'd have to not be my natural self. Wearing or getting a sew-in is one thing, but having to wear a COMPLETE wig was another. By the grace of God, I didn't really struggle with self-esteem due to this, because my mother constantly made sure we all knew we were loved and extraordinarily awesome, but I did.

In 2019, a series of events took place leading to a change in my relationship status, requiring me to do an overall rebuild. I felt that in this transitioning season as I began to rebuild certain parts of my life, everybody was going to have to get used to seeing me bald. I did a photoshoot with all my naturalness and posted it on social media January 1, 2020. I wasn't looking for approval, likes, shares, comments, support, or any of that! I just wanted people to know moving forward, that they were gonna get this bald head, and they needed to start accepting that like "Now!" LOL. Well, the response was astronomical. With thousands of likes, shares, and comments, I was blown away. Many encouraged me to not wear wigs and just be my natural self. As the days went on, I began to

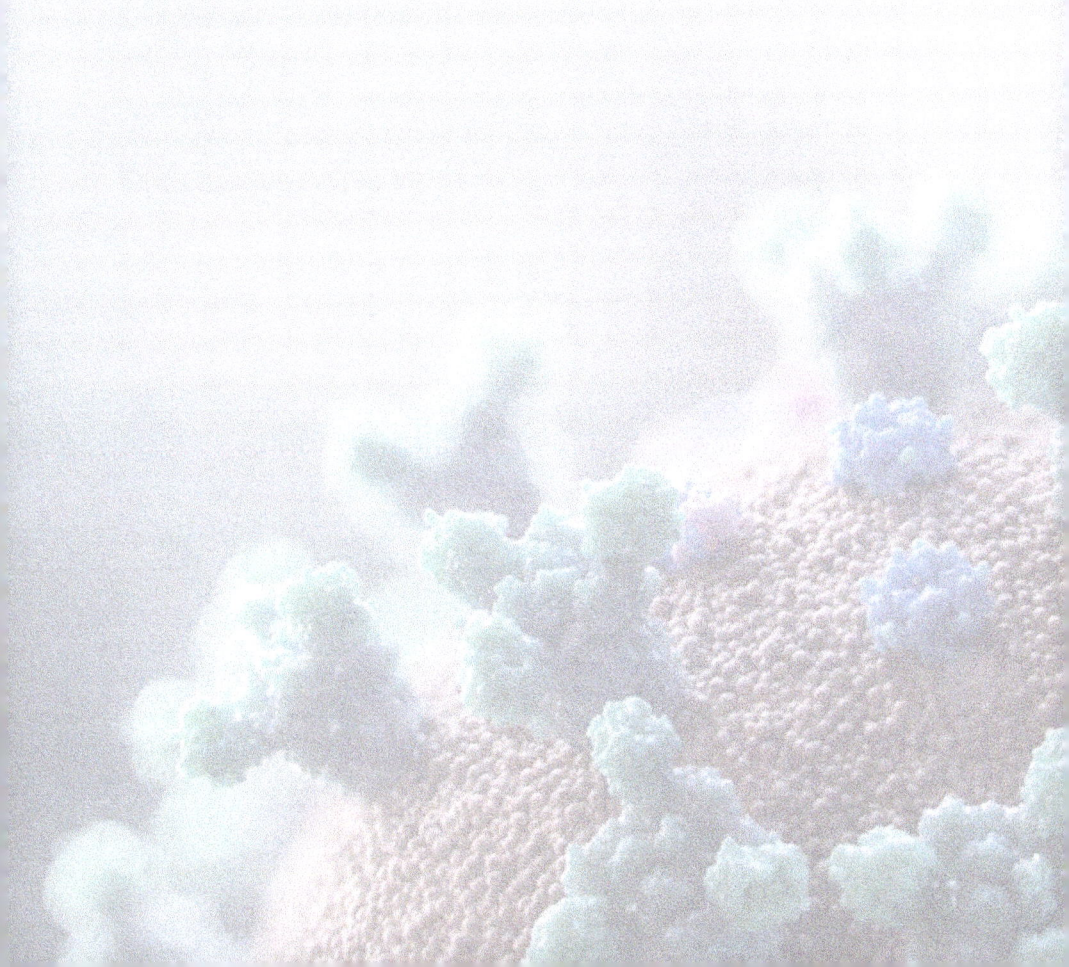

fall in love and be super comfortable with myself. The last time I wore a wig was when the Pandemic hit in March 2020.

I will be honest, I didn't know how dating would be, but to my surprise, men like bald women. LOL. Like A LOT of men. This journey of self-discovery has been exceptional. I've made it my mission to find and connect with women all over the world that have Alopecia and continue to educate the community on this auto-immune disease, and be a support to those who are struggling on their journey. I never thought the one area of my life that I was embarrassed, ashamed, and modified about would be the one thing that many love and appreciate about me. I guess it was God's plan all along!

Lorna Mastin

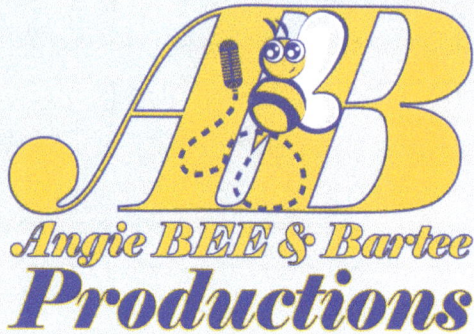

From the beginning, we knew this volume would spread Alopecia Awareness and encourage others that are facing hair loss. We also knew that we wanted to help raise funds for a non-profit organization by releasing this audiobook. The Lord heard our cry and pointed us in the direction of The Baldie Movement!   With over nine thousand followers (9,000) on Facebook alone, this social media inspiration is a powerhouse! The Baldie Movement and its founder "Nellie Nell" truly deserve our support!

A portion of the proceeds raised by Angie BEE Productions on the audiobook volume will be donated to The Baldie Movement.

This next new author truly labored over her contribution; she really just struggled as to how to get her story from her head onto paper. Our team understood completely, so we invited her to submit her story by video. Once received, our expert transcriptionist "Sonya Bee" took Shay's words from the video and added them to paper. Now, you will hear her story, in her own voice!

SLAY AS YOU ARE

Shay

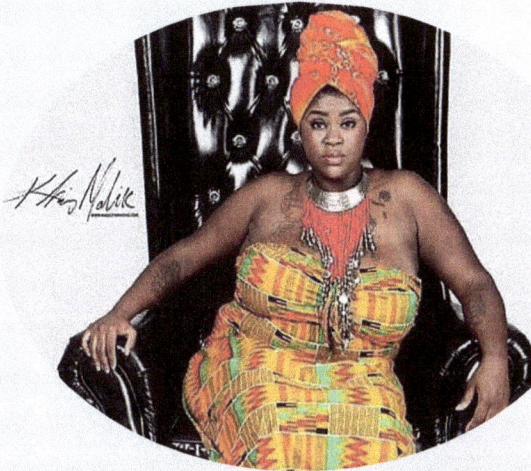

Hello, my name is Shay, and I am currently a hair stylist in Sacramento, California. I wanted to briefly share a little bit about my hair-loss journey. Unfortunately, you can't see it right now, but I lost my edges like most women. My journey of hair loss started when I was in high school – probably as early as middle school. Back in time, I received a perm at a very young age probably five, if not six, but I remember being young, and that started a process of me getting older and believing that I needed to perm my hair in order for it to be straight – not realizing that I was removing the natural coil of my hair. With that, I used to wear very tight braids, very tight singles. Literally, I had the motto, "If it wasn't tight, it wasn't right." Then eventually, I was introduced to hair-bonding glue "black glue", as we all know, for bonding tracks. As time went by, my not properly caring for it, my not properly being taught how to remove it, caused me to lose my edges and things.

I decided to want to be a hair stylist because as I got older and started to learn and study my craft, I realized there were so many women that I've connected with that suffer from the same condition that I have and who have lost confidence in this process. I believe that doing hair has given me the ability to connect with many different women on many different levels and has helped me to build a certain level of confidence within myself to be able to connect and share my own story of how I lost my edges and how I lost a lot of self-esteem behind it.

My goal, as I get deeper into my business, I will be launching a hair line the beginning of next year that's called, *Slay As You Are*. Eventually, I hope to be able to educate a lot of women on the self-esteem part of having hair loss. Even though my hair is done right now because I am a hair stylist, I have many times gone live on social media and things of that nature in my natural to let other women know, "Hey, you're not alone. Hey, that doesn't make you a bad person." Just back in time, we were not educated on certain things which resulted in losing hair. Eventually, I want to make wigs for women who have suffered from hair loss whether it be cancer, whether it be Alopecia, or all the other things that make women lose their hair. I want to be able to connect with them and make wigs and offer my services because I do believe when you have your hair done, it gives you the confidence you need.

I didn't realize that not only are young girls are suffering from it, but many adult women. I didn't realize that until I really started getting into my craft of doing hair; I learned a lot about women. Men suffer from it, but I am a woman, so I will address the womanly issue of confidence. I did not realize how many people and clients whose hair I have done were so ashamed to show who they were. Many times, my clients, who really know me, know that I'm quick to pull off their wigs if it's loose, and I can take it off to show them, "Hey, you're still beautiful; you're not your hair."

So, in saying that, I hope that my being able to share a little bit of myself and my journey will help other women to accept who they are, and if not, reach out to me and we can connect and network. We need it.

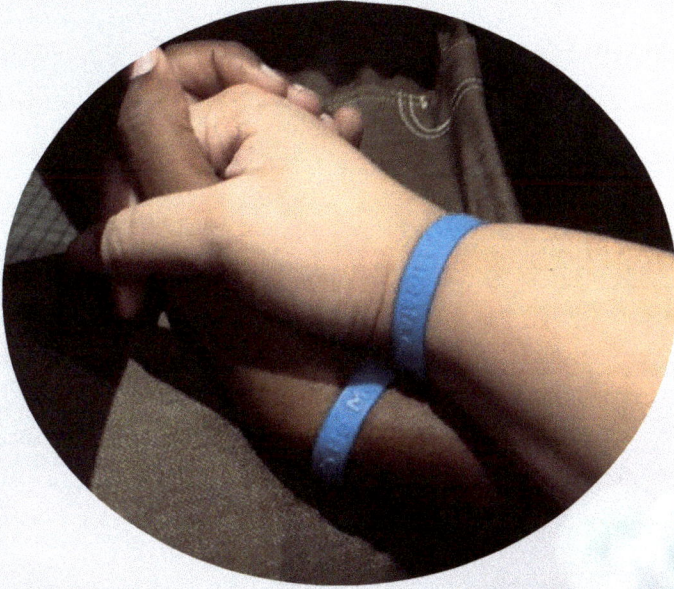

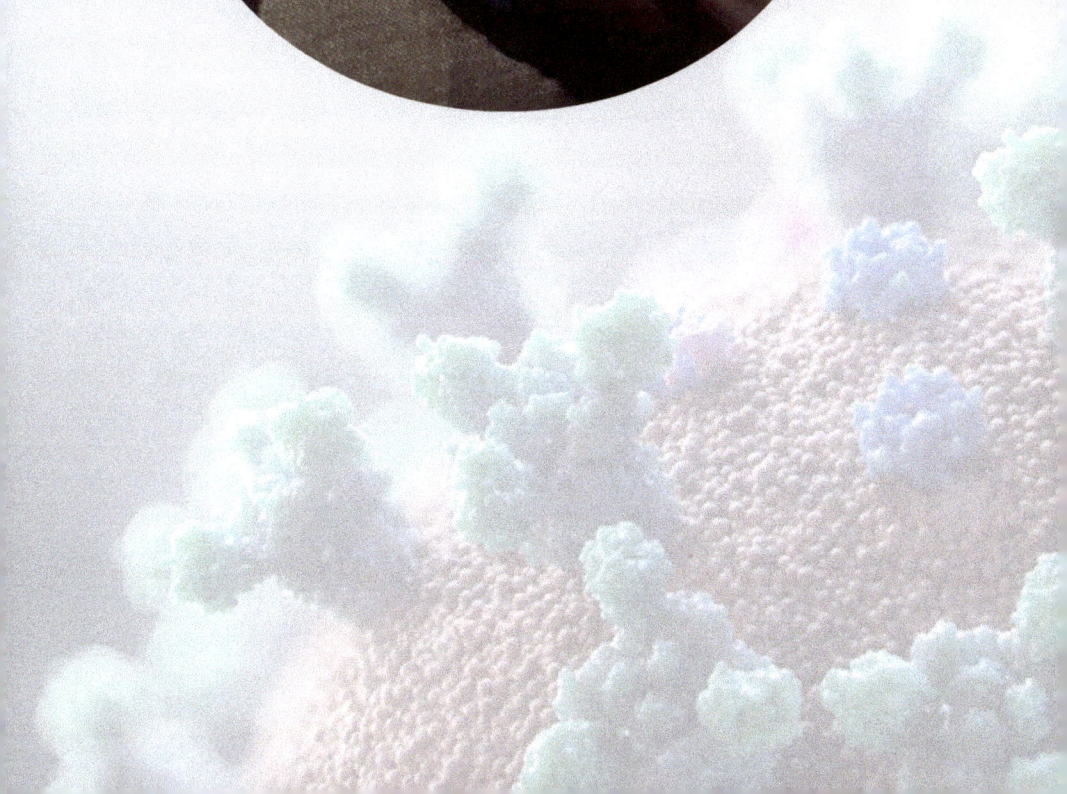

No Bad Hair Days

Uniqua Leak

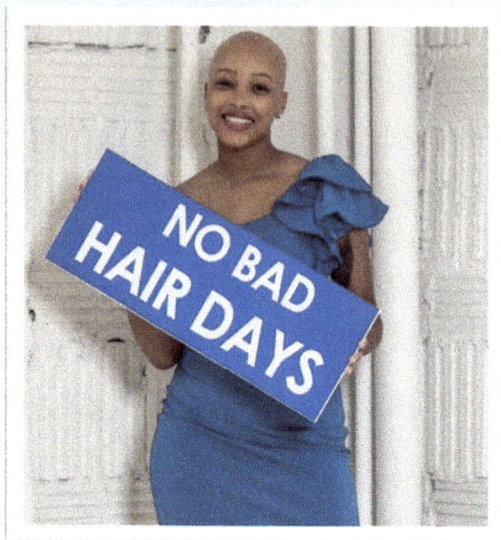

I am Uniqua Leak from Detroit, Michigan, and I have been living with Alopecia for twenty-three years. I was six years old when round-like patches of my hair began to come out. At this time, I really did not understand what was happening, and this did not immediately have an effect on me. I still had a good length of hair: it was thick, curly, and my hair stylist was able to cover the bald spots with various different styles. My grandmother wanted to find out the cause for my hair loss. I went to a number of dermatologists and cosmetologists. After being diagnosed with Alopecia Areata, I was told that the onset of my alopecia was caused from stress or trauma.

I began exploring different treatments. There was a topical cream which is a cream I applied twice daily to the bald areas on my scalp. There was an electric scalp stimulator tool for natural hair growth. None of these treatments seemed to help. Hair would grow in areas where it once was bald, but I would lose hair in other spots on my head. I got older, kids got meaner, treatments got higher in cost, and my hair began to come out faster. It was suggested that I try a more invasive treatment, known as Corticosteroid Injections. As a grade-school child I was unwilling to undergo such an invasive procedure because this involved injections on my scalp.

After having my second child in 2010, my hair rapidly began to shed. There were only two spots on opposite sides of my head where I still had hair. I was nineteen years old, and I had seen dozens of dermatologists. I was angry that treatments did not help in the past, so I decided to allow my child's father to help me shave the hair that was left on my head. I showered, combed my hair, and braided it into two different braids. We stood in the mirror of the bathroom, and as I began to cry, he shaved one braid off, and I lost all control of my emotions. I didn't let him shave the last braid. I kicked him out of the bathroom while screaming and crying. After what seemed to be hours, but more like thirty-to-forty-five minutes, I looked into the mirror and cut off the last braid. I wanted to hold on to the last braid. I found a small gold empty jewelry box. I placed both braids into the box to keep forever. This chapter is called "Shit Just Got Real."

I had to come up with a plan. I had no hair on my head for the first time in my life! What was I going to do? WIGS! I did not wear wigs or weaves when I had hair. This chapter I call, "My Frenemy." You know? You do not really like her, but you deal with her. It was a love-hate relationship. My aunt suggested I rock the bald look. When others would suggest this, it would make me angry, and I would tell them, "If you think it looks good, then shave your head and you rock it." The chemicals used in weaves and wigs did not agree with my skin. My face would break out. I tried wearing a lace front wig which had to be applied with hair glue and tape. Morgan (my first wig) was a 14-inch body wave curl. I wore her for a few months. Getting her reapplied became costly. I decided to learn to make my own wigs; I turned to You Tube. As time went on, and with a lot of practice, I got really good at this process. I grew comfortable with wearing wigs. I always wore only one style, shoulder length, blondish brown and curly. Same style I had before losing all my hair.

If not having hair on my head wasn't stressful and depressing enough, I began to lose my eyebrows. This chapter I call, "Seriously, Was the Hair on my Head Not Enough?" I honestly did not think this would be so hard on me. I was a pretty good artist. I loved to paint and draw, so I thought I could draw some eyebrows. LOL. I was so wrong. I could never draw two that looked the same. I was not a fan of having to draw on eyebrows several times a day.

Friends and family would ask all the time, "Why don't you wear your real hair anymore?" This would bother me. I did not want to explain that I have an autoimmune disease and my body is attacking my hair follicles. In 2017, I did just that! I decided to take to Facebook to reach a larger number of people. I posted two photos. One with my homemade curly wig and the other of myself with no wig. People that I have known most of my life commented in surprise, not knowing that I had been battling with hair loss. Others applauded my courage to share something so personal with the world. I cried while reading every comment. I felt like I had freed myself from this box that was sealed for so long.

As a result of my Facebook post, I was introduced to microblading, a tattooing technique that was a game changer for my "Slay, Sis" chapter. Microblading helped with my confidence greatly. I no longer needed to spend hours drawing brows on my face. The tattoos looked so natural, and I was happy.

The following year in 2018, I learned how to do headwraps. That April, I decided to put all of the weaves, glue, wigs, and head caps in the trash. I was done wearing fake hair. My twenty-seventh birthday was coming up; I had a trip planned to soak up the sun on the beach of Mexico. I arrived wearing a head scarf. Once it was time to hit the beach, the headwrap came off. I felt free! There was no one there that I knew. I told myself, "These people do not know you, so who cares if they stare!" There was a lot of staring, and I did not care. This is "Free."

The biggest test I had ahead of me was returning home to face my peers. My confidence grew. I went everywhere rocking my bald head. I received compliments all the time.

These last two years, I have chosen to love myself fearlessly. I am never looking back!

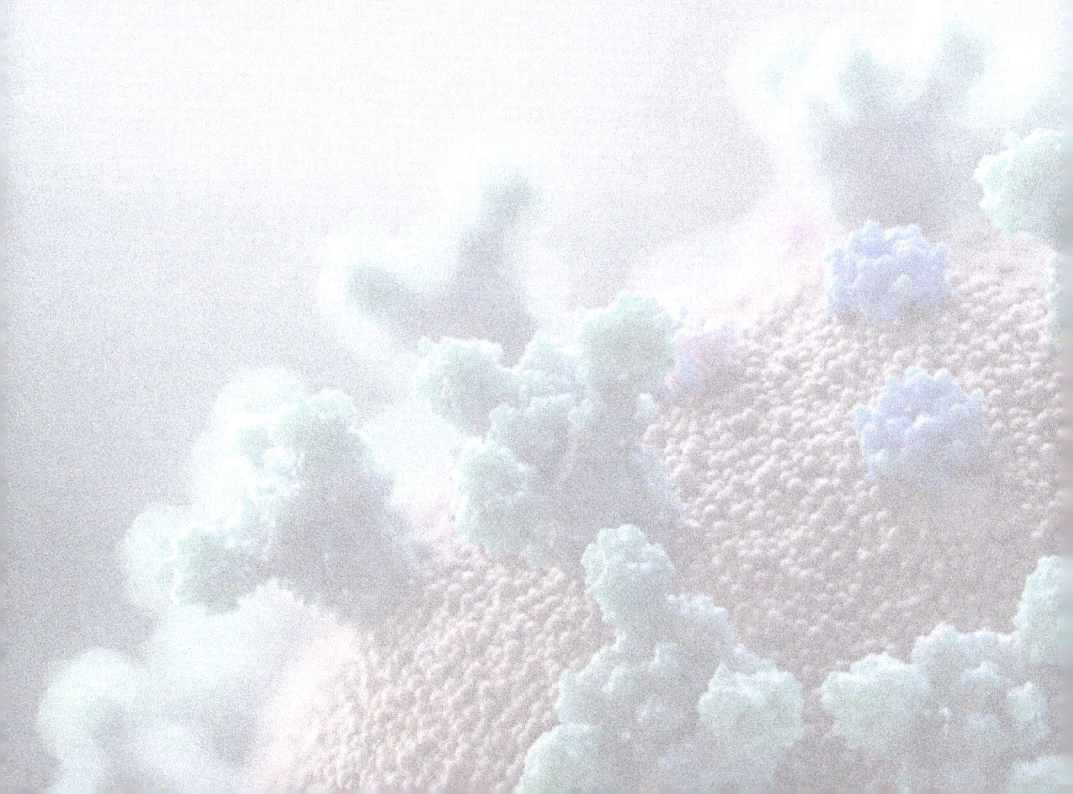

MY ALOPECIA SHORT STORY …

Tamara R. Flake

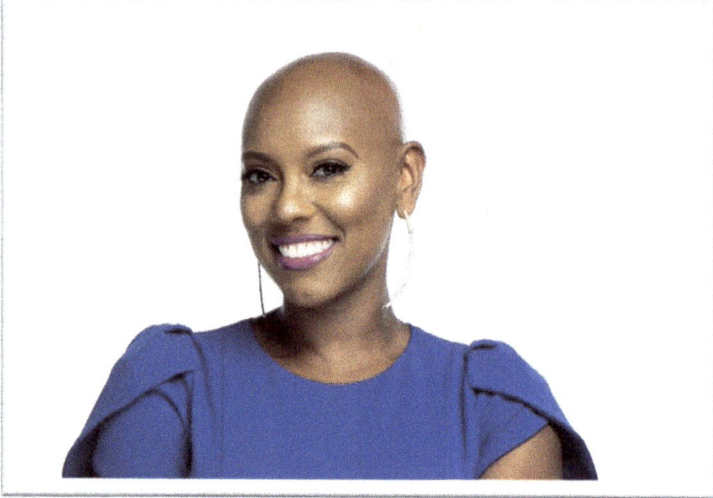

At the age of six, I began to develop dime- and quarter-sized bald spots on my head, and my parents had no idea why. See, I thought it was because I cut my hair one time in first grade with the not-so-sharp scissors they gave us in school. My parents scheduled me an appointment with the dermatologist, and that is when I was diagnosed with Alopecia Areata. Between the ages of six to twenty-nine, alopecia was a constant thought and struggle for me. I was always thinking of a way to hide my baldness under wigs, hats, headwraps and weaves. Alopecia Areata makes it difficult to wear your own hair in many stages because you experience random bald patches of all sizes throughout your head. So, I was obsessed with keeping my secret, even though it was blatantly obvious that the hair on my head was not mine, and I was clearly wearing a wig or weave. As I grew older, I was more conscious of making the wigs and weaves look more natural which was extremely expensive, but worth it to me, to avoid the stares, embarrassment, and questions.

As a kid in the 80s, it was tough wearing wigs because I did not have all the wig options that are available for kids today. I wanted so badly to wear cornrows, box braids, and ponytails, but my only options were wigs from the beauty supply store made for adult women. I was afraid to participate in sports, water activities, and anything physical for fear of my wig coming off. The only thing securing the wig to my head was the stretch band inside of it, which was not very secure at all. There was no glue or tape available back then to secure the hair to my head, and I lived in constant fear of being exposed if the wig came off, or if God forbid, someone snatched it off my head, which did happen when I was thirteen.

Fast forward to adulthood . . . I thought not having hair would hold me back from advancing professionally. It was still a process to stop wearing my wigs to work even though I had been bald in my personal life for three years before. It was liberating to stop hiding at work because it was the final step to fully embracing my truth. I had been building up to it for months. Setting dates and breaking them. For example, one time, I said my New Year's resolution would be to go to work without my wig on. THAT DIDN'T HAPPEN!! I realized I was still holding on to fear and shame of who I really was. So, I began to educate my staff, business partners, and clients about alopecia and tell them my story. I would show them pictures of me without hair to gauge their reactions. I was doing all of this to build up my courage to come to work without the hair and to gain their support whenever I decided to do so.

Support is important to have through this process. I have always had a strong support system with my family. So, in my mind, I needed the support of my work family to get through this next phase in my journey. Finally, on April 23, 2012 (thanks for the memory Facebook), I DID IT! I went to work without my hair. I made sure my makeup was on point, and I was dressed really cute and professionally with the perfect accessories. I walked in that building with my head high and an attitude that said, "I am strong. I am Bold. I am courageous. I am beautiful. I AM UNAPOLOGETICALLY ME!"

Alopecia was once something that I was ashamed of having; however, when I felt that way, it was because I wanted to be like everyone else. That time, between ages six and twenty-nine, was a major growth phase for me. It took time for me to learn who Tamara truly is. It was a process ... a journey that I needed to experience to arrive at my authenticity. Now, I LOVE that Alopecia makes me different! I stand out, and I am not like anyone else. I have a story to share to empower and encourage someone who needs to hear it. Alopecia has freed me to be my true authentic self, and that is a woman I can be proud of! I do not hide; I am not afraid; I live life to the fullest and embrace every experience without fear of being exposed and embarrassed. I took my power back. I am uniquely me, and I would not trade me for anyone else in the world!

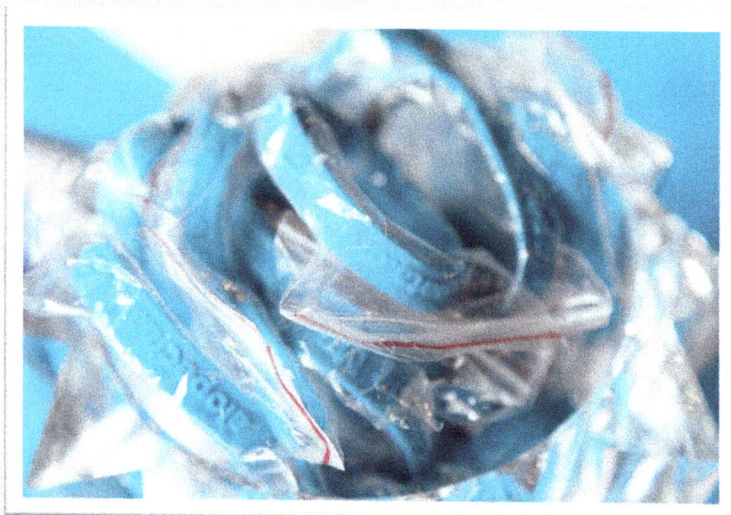

Photo by Jhonn de la Puente
www.facebook.com/jdlpphotography

THE STORY OF BOLD AND BALDNESS

Raquel Johnson

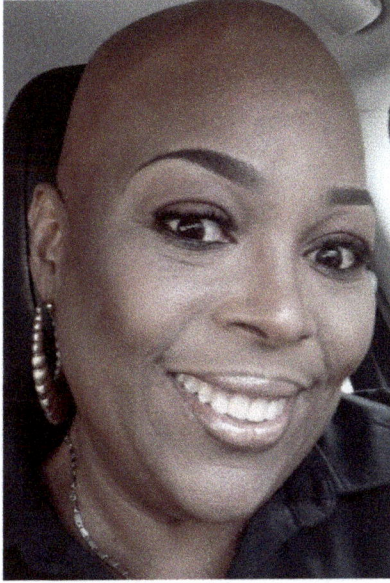

I grew up in Detroit, Michigan, where I come from a family of cosmetologists and barbers. My dad was a licensed Cosmetologist/Barber whose primary focus was healthy hair. He owned his own barber shop on Harper and Dickerson named Exodus. Having three children, two girls and boy, and my mother, who was the wife, it was my dad's responsibility to provide haircare for his family.

My hair was long, super thick, and hard to manage. I can remember my dad performing electro treatments, specialized conditions, and constant brushing, along with massaging my scalp and my mother's, as well. He took great pride in growing my hair until his untimely passing at the age of thirty-three. I was only ten years old when my father went to sleep and died as a result of a brain aneurysm. My hair continued to grow and grow. The thickness and texture were so strong. I was always told by beauticians that I had a good head of hair to work with.

I am fifty years old today. In my thirties, which was in the 2000s, I noticed that my hair began to thin out in such a way that I was forced to wear braids or hair weave with the hopes of covering up those thin spots. Well, the covering up only lasted for so long. My hair began to come out around the frontal part of my head and in the center. I was about thirty-six years old when I made my first appointment to see a dermatologist. It was then I was told by my doctor that I had alopecia. My doctor began to tell me about treatments, which were the injections that I began to hate so badly. After a few years of constantly going to see the dermatologist and getting those awful painful injections that did not help my situation, I began to become more frustrated day by day. At that point in my life, I began to buy human hair and get full hair weaves that were sewed onto French braids. Ohhh! I thought this was the lifetime fix. Something I could afford and looked nice, and no one knew about the severe thinning underneath. After four-to-five years of wearing weaves/sew-ins, my hair began to fall out all around the front and in the top. I was no longer able to get a regular weave. It was that day when I began to follow this young man name Richard Anthony on Facebook who was in Atlanta, Georgia.

Richard Anthony is a stylist in Atlanta who specializes in making hair units for women who suffers from alopecia. His technique is unbelievable. My mother would help finance my trips to Atlanta, Georgia, to get custom wigs made by the one and only Richard Anthony B.K.A. Prince Charming. These wigs would cost me anywhere between four hundred to seven hundred dollars. They were handmade and would last for a few years. I would wear what is called frontals or 360s. These wigs came with customized hair lines and parts throughout the wig that looks like your regular scalp. The wigs were awfully expensive until I found a young lady in Detroit named Marlene Brooks who was able to customize wigs and sew-ins, as well. I rocked those wigs and frontal sew-ins for years without many people knowing about my hair condition. At this point in my life, I was not able to grow hair anywhere but around the side. My hair was completely gone in the top and all around the front.

In 2016 to 2020, a series of events began to happen. In 2016, I lost my first cousin Tamela Wolfe to brain cancer. She was only forty-seven years old. I was devastated, and it sent me into depression. On February 10, 2018, my beautiful mother suffered a massive stroke right before my eyes as she was showing me how to use my snow blower. My mother was my everything. My mother held on at the hospital for seven days and transitioned on February 17. I was broken and did not know how to move forward without her. I did the work and attended grief counseling, and I also participated in a support grief support. On March 25, 2020, during COVID-19, I lost my only brother whose name was Orlando Johnson. He suffered a massive heart attack; they think he may have also had COVID-19. The medical examiner stated that he had pneumonia, but they did not give him a test for COVID-19 because he expired in the ambulance. My brother's death sent me back into depression.

My sister and I laid my brother away as we knew my mom would want us to. It was at this point where I had just had enough! I never wanted to disclose the fact that I had alopecia. My brother's daughter was angry with me and my sister after my brother passed. My family has always been close and stuck together with each other. My niece threatened to disclose my baldhead on Facebook. I panicked; I did not know what to do. I was so angry because I did not want anyone to know that I suffered from alopecia. A few days later, I made the decision to shave my hair off and acknowledge that I am an alopecia survivor. My reveal on Facebook was overwhelming. I received over five hundred-plus positive posts. I thank God for allowing me to reveal my bald head and tell my story.

My name is Raquel Johnson, and I have survived Alopecia.

THERE'S BEAUTY IN YOUR FLAWS

A Poem by Shay

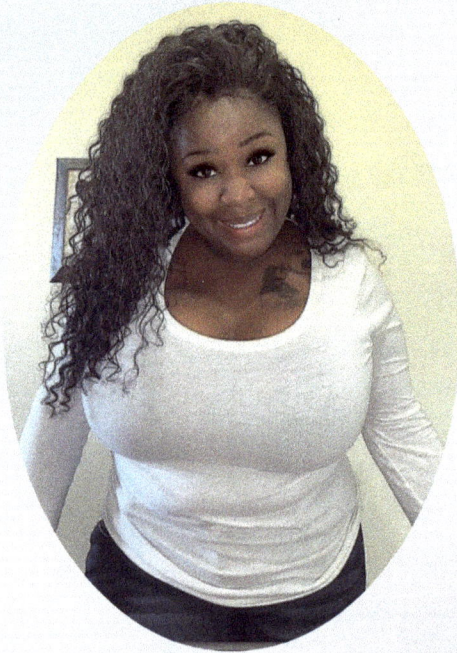

What does it mean to be beautiful you see that's now the answer I seek because growing up I always thought beauty was considered skin deep way past what the eyes could see yet you see I'm standing here all dolled up in pretty still seeking the definition of beauty I got all my eyelashes I even painted on my face an' dang can you believe I even found something to slim down my waist trying to fit into what society sees as the perfect beauty and can you believe it I even want that bigger booty so I looked at some channels flip through some shows on TV and then ask myself is this who I really want to be because this is what people see as reality no no that most definitely ain't me but just sit back and relax as I flip to the next chapter and show you a different form of me let's just called this next chapter the purist form of the real and natural me.

Well, here I am just as natural as can be the realist form of natural ol' me so tell me do I now fit in now that I've uncovered the real me now that I've showed you as natural as I can be. No edges no make up my lace front now gone but don't make me feel like I did some kind of wrong. You see it's time we learn to realize that this too is beauty it's just what you would call a real natural beauty so let's not throw shade on another sister's flaws because truth be told we all got some kind of flaw, some choose to Hide it while others stand tall but sista I'm here to help u to learn to embrace them all. So love yourself and don't be afraid to be free and if and when you do always remember this is the natural ol' me.

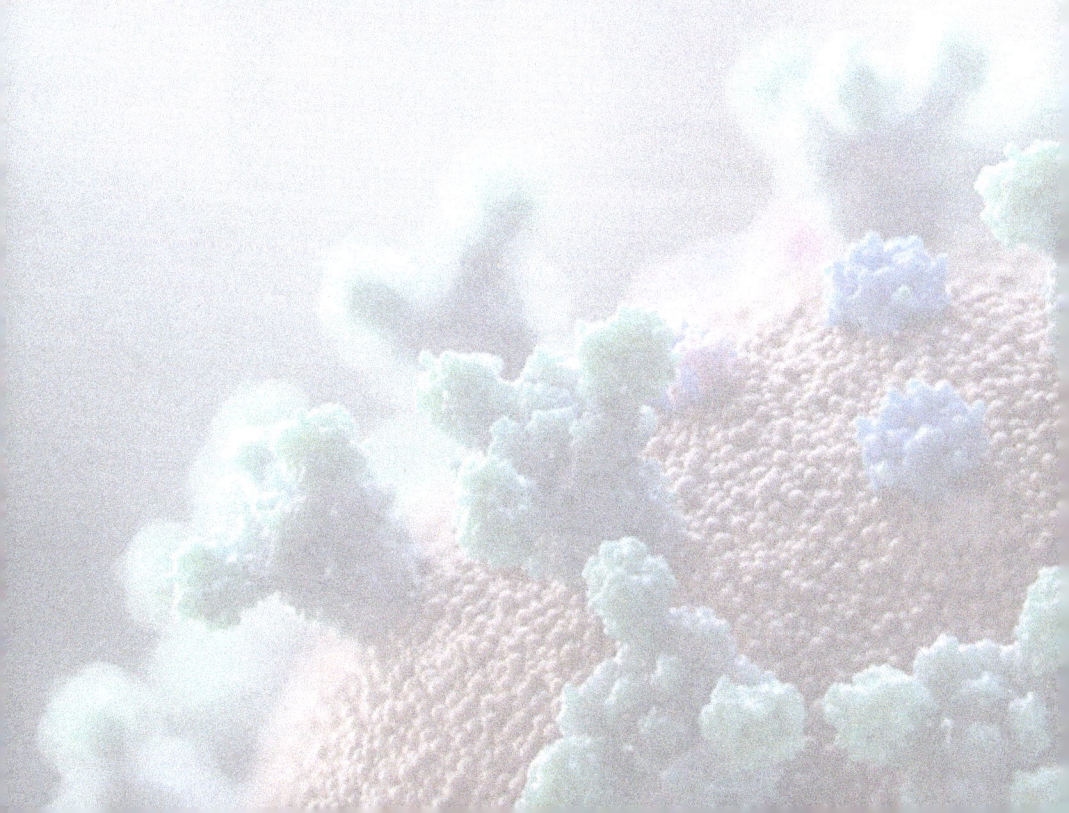

212 | COMPILED BY ANGIE BEE & BARTEE PRODUCTIONS

How Can I NOT Like a Bold, Beautiful and Bald Woman?

Bartee

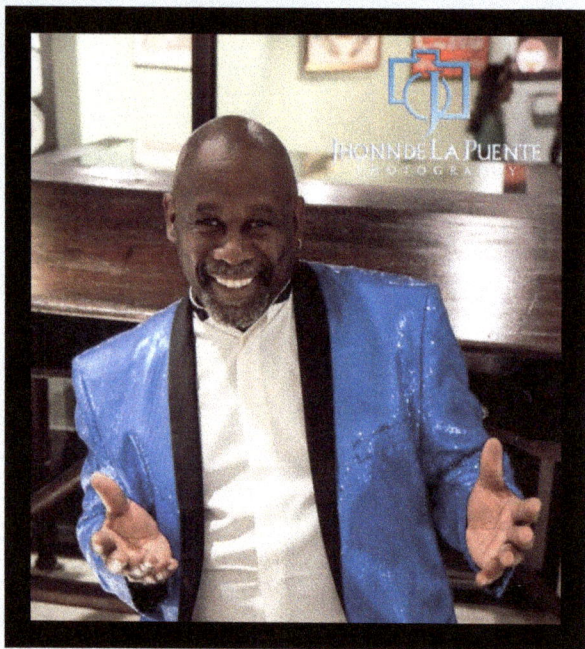

You know, after listening to some jazz music, I told Angela that she had some pretty lips. I asked her if I could kiss her. Her response was (I really don't remember what she said), but anyway, we kissed! After sitting down and talking with each other about matters of the heart, Angela explained to me that she had a mental illness, and we talked about that for a while. Then, she took off her wig and explained to me that she had Alopecia (although I didn't know what that meant at the time).

First of all, let me state that she looked like a "China Baby" with her smooth, clear, shiny bald head. I kinda smiled because I didn't see any knots or bumps or hills to climb (LOL!), if you know what I mean. So, with that, I was good!

Now, it would have been another story if her head wasn't as smooth and shaped like a China Baby! And you know, knowing me, I would have told her, "Hey, you know, maybe you need to keep that wig on and maybe cut it down a little bit" because her wig was kinda long and thick, and I knew it was a wig in the first place (LOL).

Everyone is not as fortunate to have a nice round scalp for a bald head, so one must have enough confidence in themselves to wear that type of look – that Baldie Look! So, to say what I need to say, "Be Bold, Beautiful and Bald!"

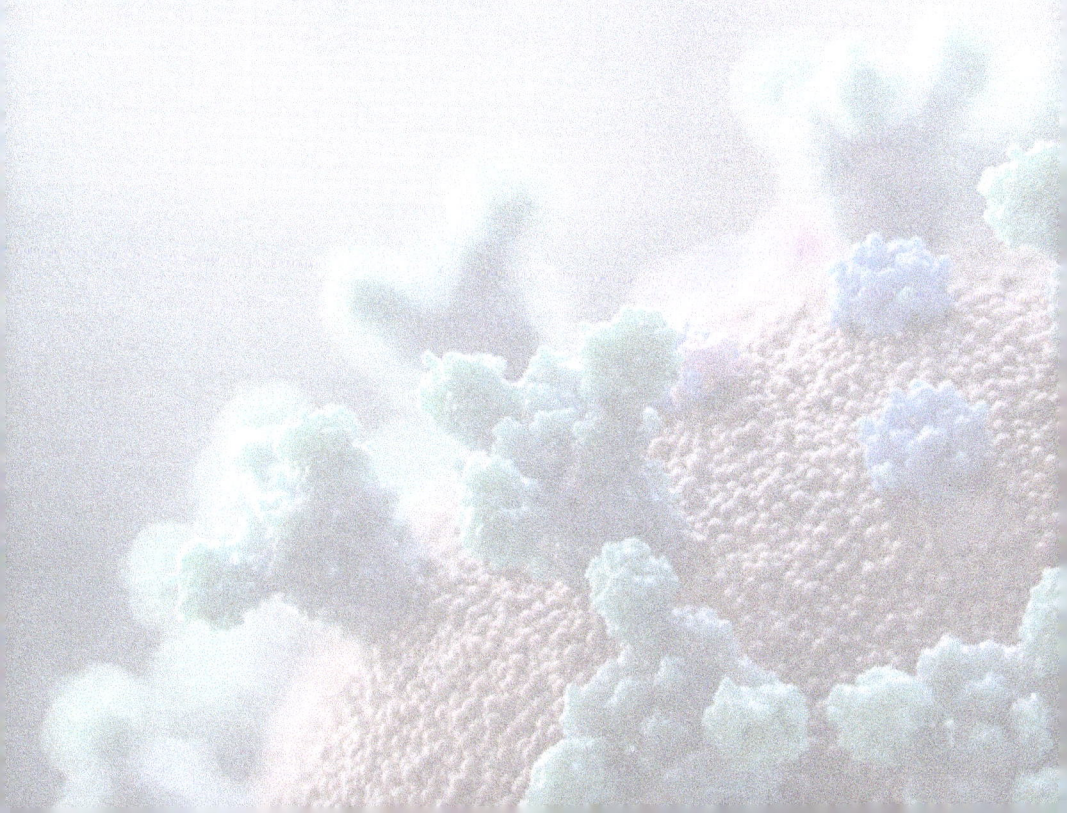

My Story

Evangelist Angie BEE

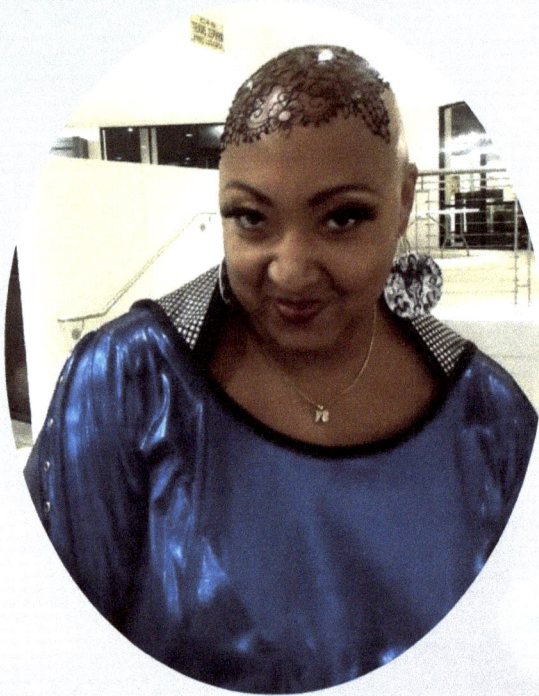

This photo was taken at the 2019 Bold Beautiful & Bald Beauty Bazaar in Daytona Beach, Florida.

My gown and cape were created by Senia Soto of Jarix Designs. My earrings were created by Arlene Hall-Scarlett, CEO of Novyedesigns.

Tiffany Tyson Green of Sophisticated Tips adorned me with my eyelashes, and my henna "crown" came from one of our event vendors.

My contribution was originally printed in the September 2020 issue of *Triumphant Magazine*. This inspirational publication has featured our *Confinement Chronicles* authors each month since we first launched our audiobook series. Search for *Triumphant Magazine* on Facebook and tell publisher Theresa Jordan that we are so grateful for her support. This is My Story.

September is Alopecia Awareness Month, so if you begin to see a lot of royal blue images everywhere, that is because men, women, and children just like me are celebrating and sharing what we live with as Alopecians!

Although I preach, speak, lead workshops, and appear on Facebook LIVE each week with my bald head glistening, people still ask me, *"Angie BEE, why are you bald? Don't you want to try a wig to cover your head? Are you sick? Are you having treatments? Would you like to try this and that to make your hair grow?"*

So, let's have a conversation. According to the National Alopecia Areata Foundation at www.NAAF.org, *"Alopecia areata is a common autoimmune skin disease, causing hair loss on the scalp, face and sometimes on other areas of the body. In fact, it affects as many as 6.8 million people in the U.S. with a lifetime risk of 2.1%"*. I unknowingly started showing signs of this disease in 1995. My then-hairdresser offered to glue in a weave to cover the bald patches that she saw. I didn't see them, and she wanted to try something new, so I agreed to it! Not long after that, my daughters and I were in a head-on collision with an 18-wheel semi-tractor, pulling a trailer. During my recovery, as my mother was combing my hair, she immediately recognized my bald spaces.

"Angie, you have Alopecia. My dermatologist diagnosed me with a form of it too," my mother told me.

In 2017, Donna Gray-Banks encouraged me and Bartee to launch an annual event that allows those with alopecia to gather together in a social and informative session to learn and network. The Bold Beautiful & Bald Beauty Bazaar debuted as a one-day shopping and fashion event in Daytona Beach, Volusia County, Florida. Each year the event has doubled in size, and in 2018, we even added a Weekend Beachside Retreat! Fashion show models, sponsors, guests, and friends gather at a designated host resort and enjoy evening s'mores, photo shoots, a dinner boat cruise, workshops, and fellowship. Last year, we learned how to apply magnetic eyelashes (when you have no eyelashes or eyebrows, this is an important class to have). The year prior, we learned about financing, marriage and relationship tips from Author Kayl May (Atlanta), and "Stan the State Farm Insurance Man" Stan Harrison of New Smyrna Beach, Florida. **There were even two lovebirds that attended our 2018 weekend retreat relationship workshop, and now they are married! One of them has alopecia and the other one doesn't care. They see each other for who they are and how God brought them together!** They are BLESSED!

The next time you see a bald person, don't stare, don't frown, don't whisper, or turn away. Give us a BIG smile and a THUMBS UP because you don't know the journey it took for us to snatch off those wigs and flaunt our beautiful bald heads!

Learn more about our annual Alopecia Awareness weekend event at www.daqueenbee.com/boldbeautifulandbald and follow us at www.Facebook.com/BoldBeautifulAndBaldBeautyBazaar

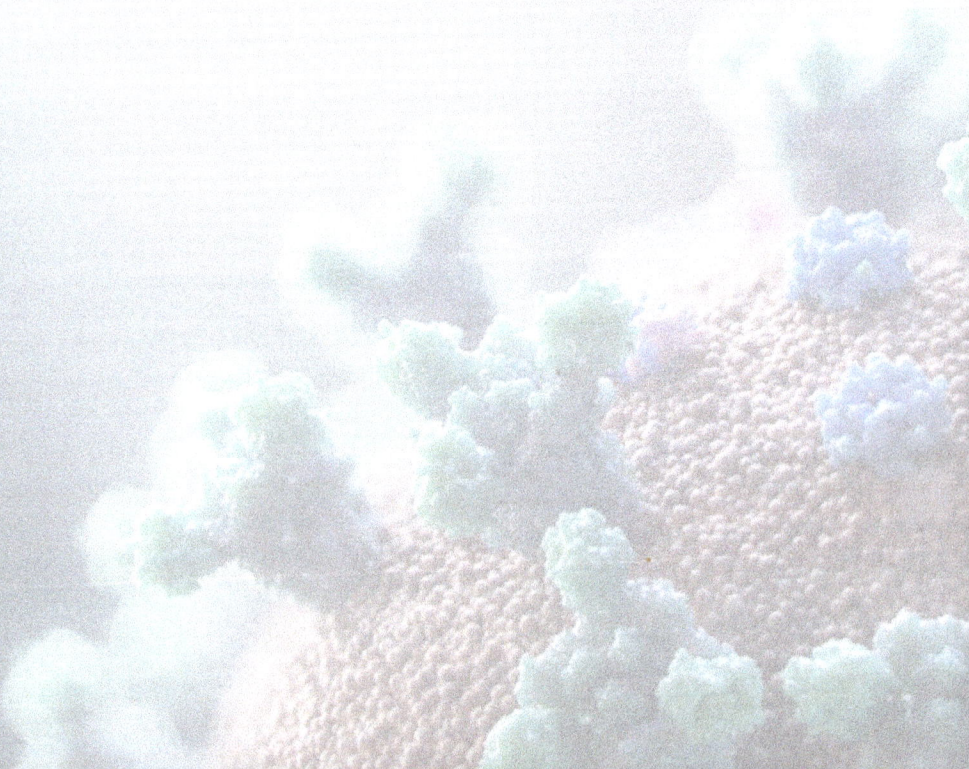

Sometimes, an author needs to speak his/her words using a video camera or a recorder. Afterwards, a true talent like SONYA BENNETT can transcribe those words, and even include the correct punctuation, all in print. A very special thank you to Sonya for transcribing the video submitted to this project. Thank you for helping me to capture and include those words in this issue of *Confinement Chronicles*.

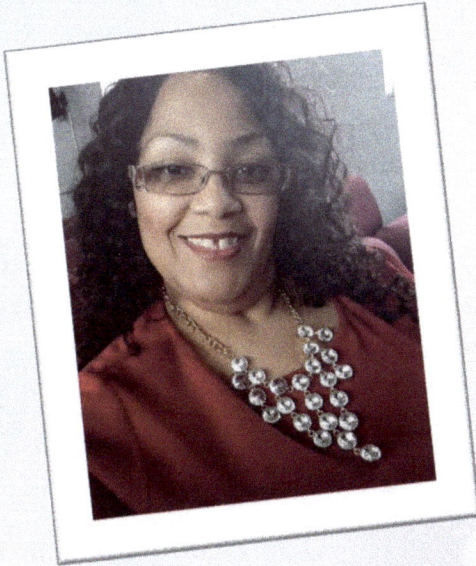

Sonya Bennett
Professional Transcriptionist with Angie BEE Productions

This concludes *Confinement Chronicles* and the #IrefuseToStopBeingMe volume, which serves as a fundraiser for The Baldie Movement. A portion of the proceeds from this project were donated to this 501C3-non-profit organization, and we invite YOU to make a donation, too. Please visit www.TheBaldieMovement.org to learn more and to show your support.

Thank you to "Da Bee Hive Intern Crew" at Angie BEE Productions. I would also like to thank my family for assisting me with the completion of this project; especially my beloved husband Bartee. Not only did he assist with me narration and sponsor commercial production, but he loves me unconditionally with, or without hair. Thank you, Bartee!

These stories shall continue!

Follow ConfinementChroniclesByAngieBEEproductions on Facebook.

Be safe and BEE Blessed

Sincerely,

Evangelist Angie BEE

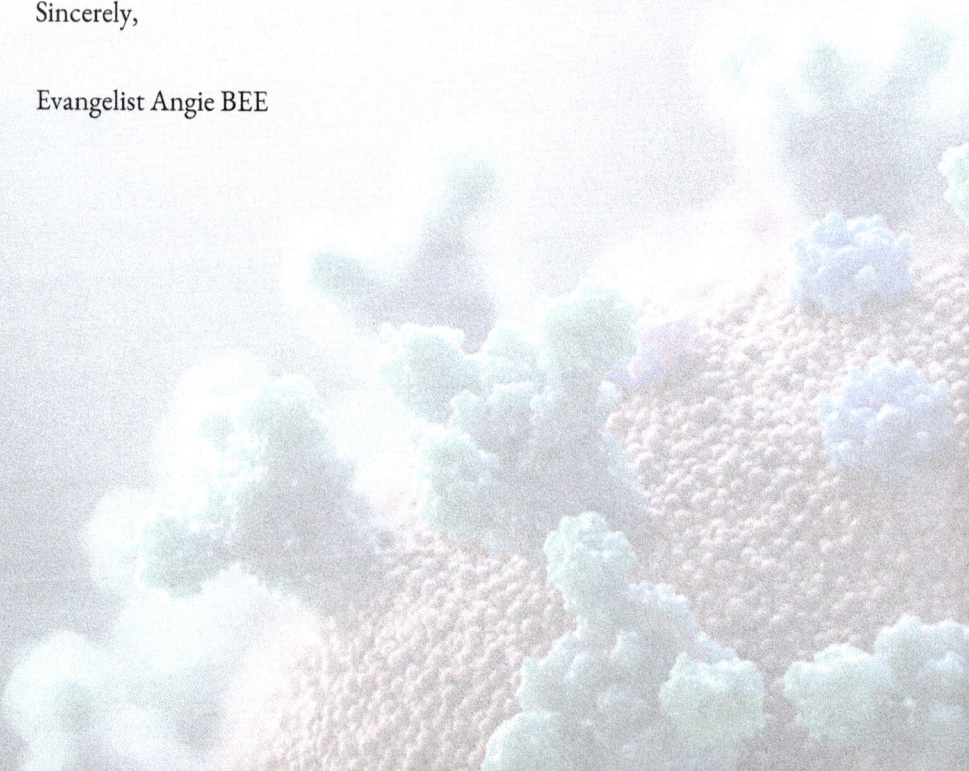

VOLUME X

Confinement Chronicles Surviving COVID

Even In My Darkness hour...

YOU NEVER LEFT ME

Psalm 18:19

An inspirational audiobook compilation series produced by

ANGiE Bee Productions
Ministry, media and more

Volume X

I t is Monday morning, October 19, 2020, the opening day of early voting in several counties in Florida. My husband and I are standing in the line, outside of the library in Daytona Beach, Florida. We couldn't wait for the weekend to end! "We are going to vote on Monday!" "We are going to vote tomorrow!!" I said to Bartee. Each time I mentioned voting, he had a smile on his face; he was pretty excited, too.

The line was so long outside the election location that several election volunteers walked up to us to hand us pamphlets. Bartee and I once served on a re-election committee for a local judge, so we realize how the volunteers feel when you reject their offer for information, so, we graciously accepted the handout and read it over. On this date, it seemed that not only were we inundated with information, but we were also surrounded by very opinionated people.

> "I don't know why I have to wear this damned mask!"
> grumbled one elderly man.

> "It's just a flu! They got us all riled up for nothing but a flu!"
> another white-haired gentleman proclaimed.

> "I just don't believe it's real. Between me and my wife,
> we've got 15 doctors, and they all say it ain't real,"
> another man interjected.

After finally having heard enough of the comments, another man, much younger than the others, turned from his place in the voting line and loudly stated:

> "I had COVID -19, and it almost killed me.
> Keep your opinions to yourself!"

The woman standing with him in line gently placed her hand on his shoulder and encouraged him to turn back around in the line. We all remained quiet for the remainder of our time "together", and I said a prayer for each person that surrounded us.

Later that evening, as I reflected on my voting experience, the Lord brought me back to this volume of the *Confinement Chronicles* series. The scripture that He assigned to this volume several months ago is Psalm 18:19. When I sat at my computer to look it up again, guess what the New International version of the bible says:

> *He brought me out into a spacious place;*
> *he rescued me because he delighted in me.*
> Psalm 18:19

I SEE YOU, GOD! You knew MONTHS ago that I would be out in a spacious place (outside the library, standing in a long line, waiting to vote). You knew MONTHS ago that on this day I would have grumbling in front of me, complaining behind me, attempted swaying on the right of me, and a fence to my left – and YOU RESCUED ME! I found peace in my mind today, in spite of all the negativity surrounding me, and I delighted myself by seeking YOU through prayer. He rescued me! I survived that situation and many, MANY other situations because the first thing I did was to pray.

I have seen people complain about the new normal after effects of the pandemic, and I have seen families DEVASTATED by this virus. This audiobook will share just a few stories with you to inform and encourage you. We ask you to pray for the individuals and families that are reflected in this project and we ask that you continue to pray for the world as we all strive to heal.

We have arrived at the final volume in this pandemic series. This is Volume X, and portions of it deal with grief, shock, and praise. COVID-19 attacked the younger and the older, those in good health and the wealthy, too. Some of us have suffered in silence, while others are still waiting for a "cure/vaccine." I am grateful for those that God has placed in my life that continue to help keep me safe during this pandemic. My husband shops for groceries and checks on my mental health; my daughters check on me DAILY as I have endured surgeries, biopsies, and healing this year. I thank God for the prescription medication that I take daily, and I thank Him for the physicians, surgeons, and other medical professionals that have cared for me in Gainesville, Daytona, and Ormond Beach, Florida.

As a mental health advocate, I continue to live with symptoms of major depression disorder, generalized anxiety disorder, and post-traumatic stress disorder while in this pandemic, so I understand how others feel at this time! I strive to share my story with others – to help educate them. Now, as the pandemic rages through our lives and our families, others are experiencing symptoms and they don't recognize them ... they feel lost and confused. It is my prayer that this audiobook and the first nine volumes in this series will help them to realize that they are not alone, and lead them to seek the help that they need.

Join me in prayer for our country. Pray with me that the bereaved are comforted and those that are ill will find help and strength from the Lord.

Share this with others!

And now, for our first contribution...

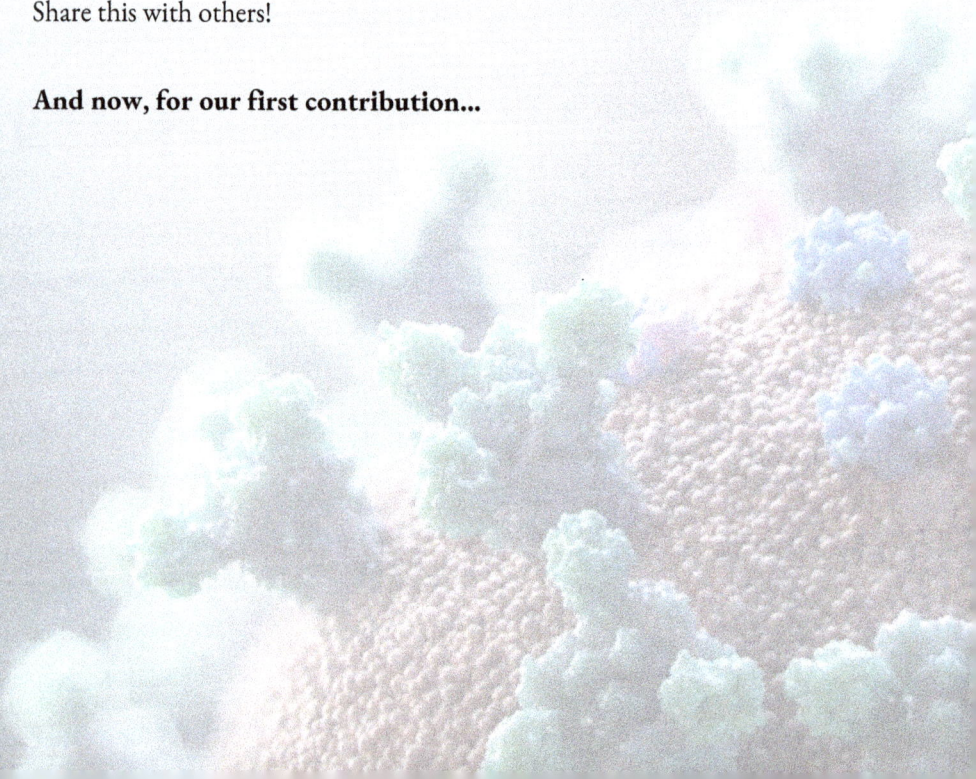

EVEN IN MY DARKEST HOUR . . . YOU NEVER LEFT ME

Theresa Jordan

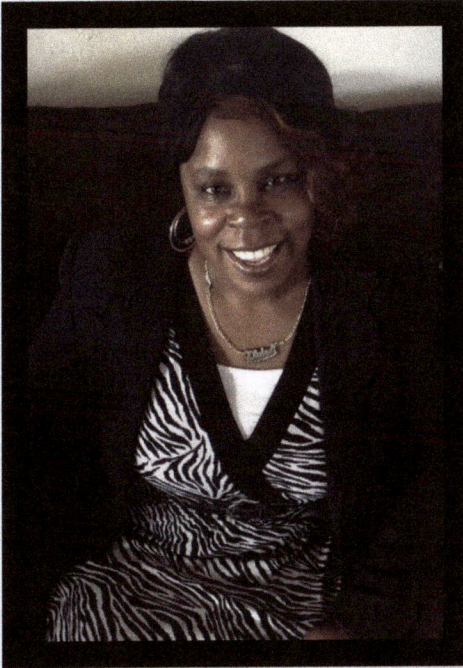

I can honestly say, "Even In My Darkest Hour the Lord has never left me, and I am so grateful." During my darkest days, He has been with me every step of the way. I can literally find traces of God's footprints working in the front and back scenes of my life. There have been several occasions in my life where the Lord showed me, "Theresa Jordan, your life is in my hands."

I found out when I was a baby that my biological father had me in his hands, and he was trying to hand me over the gate to someone, but his attempt was unsuccessful because my small infant body landed on the sidewalk of Paterson, New Jersey. I would discover this happened to me when I became an adult, and afterwards, I can recall having several conversations with my late Aunt/Mother/Friend Loretta King, and my late biological Mother Eloise Wade. I was truly a miracle baby, because I should not have been here today, and I could have been dead. But God! He has greater plans for my life, and I am so grateful. I also know this because Jeremiah 29:11-13 tells me, *For I know the thoughts that I think toward you, saith the LORD, thoughts of peace, and not of evil, to give you an expected end.*

> *12 Then shall ye call upon me, and ye shall go and pray unto me, and I will hearken unto you.*
> *13 And ye shall seek me, and find me, when ye shall search for me with all your heart.*

2015: I had to say goodbye to my Aunt Dora a.k.a. Lorretta – the hardest decision I had to make in my life. We know that this world is not a permanent home, but it is never easy saying goodbye to our loved ones.

But when I look over my life and take an inventory, I can say, "The Lord has been good to me, and He has been with me every step of the way."

2019: I never could have imagined in 2015, God was preparing me for my own mother four years later. My mother and I were like twins because we resembled each other; we wore the same size clothes; and we both have a great sense of humor. Our middle names are Determined and Resilient, and we always looked to the hills from which cometh all our help. We knew the power of praying and trusting in God's Word. As I am writing this next month, November 4th will be one year. Death is never easy, but God promised me that He would never leave me nor forsake me. But God is faithful, and He cannot tell a lie. He has kept me, and he has strengthened me through all of this, and He has strengthened me through all that. Because I know the Joy of the Lord is my Strength, and He has been my strength down through the years. God is my everything.

He has always been there to guide me through the darkest hours and moments in my life. Jesus has been there with me every step of the way, and He knows how much each of us can bear. There is a saying, "If God brings you to it, He is more than qualified to bring each of us through it." Now, I am guilty of always adding my twist to quotes, but you can understand the concept. The Lord provides me with His wisdom, understanding, and endurance everyday of my life. He is faithful because He duplicates those same attributes during my greatest moments in life.

God has blessed me to run through hoops and leap over walls according to His Word. My husband Daniel teases me frequently by saying, "Theresa, God has blessed you with several mothers". I just look at my husband, and I start laughing because he is correct with his statements. I must take full ownership of Daniel's statements because God knew what I needed to make me into the phenomenal and amazing woman that I am today. God knew what it would take to have me fully walking in my true purpose and calling. With all the above said, God has blessed me to have three beautiful, strong, intelligent, God-fearing and entrepreneurial women in my life: my Nana a.k.a. Fannie Mims, my (late) Aunt Dora, and my (late) mother Eloise Wade. The Lord knew I needed these dynamite women because they would be in the molding and shaping of my life. They would teach me through their personal experiences, struggles, challenges, and the ups and downs in life how to remain unbreakable and unstoppable. God also knew these women, by His grace, would fully equip me to have what I needed during these challengeing times we are facing in our world today. He knew by placing everything inside of me that I would be blessed, and I would be willing to pay it forward to this generation and generations to come. These three strong women He placed in my life became resilient, and they did not allow this world or anybody else to dictate what they deserved. They leaned, depended, and trusted in God's Holy Word.

My Nana was fortunate enough to celebrate her 87th birthday on June 6th. Cissy Houston is the mother of the late Whitney Houston; she also recently celebrated her 87th birthday on September 30th . The good Lord has smiled and blessed both tremendously.

I moved to Georgia with my Nana at the age of thirteen. Prior to moving, I lived in Paterson, New Jersey, but Nana decided to not become like Lot's wife . . . and that was looking back. Now, she had already raised five children of her own, and she was willing, by the grace of God, to raise me as her sixth child. But God has the master plan, and I have learned that concept from Dr. Lucille O'Neal because her mother would always remind her of this. It was nonnegotiable about finishing high school and then going to college. My Nana was willing to sacrifice everything to have me become the first out of the family to attend college and finish college. I can attest the mission was accomplished, and I am grateful God allowed my Nana to see the potential inside of me before I could see the potential inside myself.

Jekelyn Carr has a song in which she speaks haivng and experiencing greater things in life, just like the oil that results from the beating and pressing of olives.

I believe my greater is here, and I believe my greater has come. To God Be the Glory! I am expecting God to literally blow my mind during this season and the seasons to come beyond 2020. I am excited about the things the Lord has in store for me. Because the Word declares in 1 Corinthians 2:9:

But as it is written, Eye hath not seen, nor ear heard, neither have entered into the heart of man, the things which God hath prepared for them that love him.

During the season of surviving COVID-19, God continues to show me His brilliance, mercy, grace, and His impeccable and Sovereign ways. He continues to be there for me during my darkest hours, and I am grateful. I am blessed to be in a place where I fully trust the Lord because He knows what is best for me. I am reminded to reflect on the goodness of Jesus.

This is an immensely powerful song by Rev. Paul Jones, and it is called, "I Won't Complain." We are encouraged, in spite of the situations we face, to not complain for God has still been GOOD!

I am reminded of Psalm 37:25 which reads, *I have been young, and now am old; yet have I not seen the righteous forsaken, nor his seed begging bread.*

Until next time, remain safe, healthy, and encouraged in the Lord always.

MY COVID-19 EXPERIENCE

Charlene Stewart

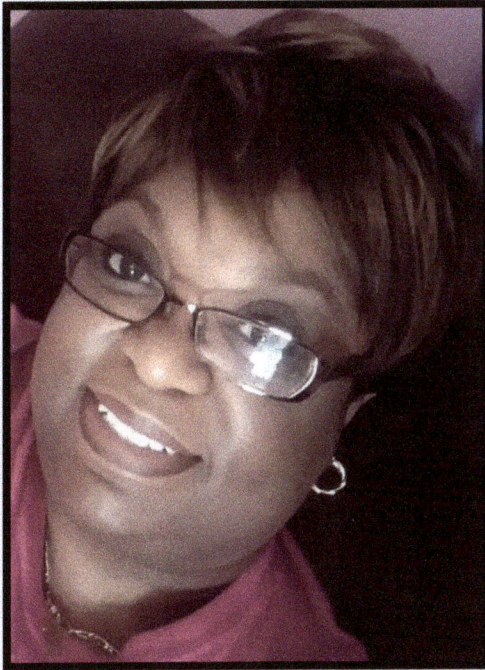

My name is Charlene! I am a wife, a mother, a friend, a neighbor, but out of all these tributes . . . I AM A SURVIVOR!!

I was not feeling well during the week of June 29th. I was experiencing body aches, a slight cough and a high fever that wouldn't go away with the use of Advil or Aleve. I virtually contacted my doctor, who instructed me to go get tested for COVID-19 in the hospital parking lot of NAS JAX, a military installation in Jacksonville, Florida.

That test was worse than giving birth! The nursing staff, manning make-shift lab in the parking lot, were administering the test while you sat idling in your car. The testing instrument, a thin plastic swab with fine soft bristles on one end and a knob to screw into a vial on the other end, was shoved up one nostril with no regard to the pain they (the nurses) were delivering. It felt as if a bug had flown up your nose and you try so desperately to blow it out to no avail.

After testing, I went home and quarantined myself in my room. I was afforded the amenities of having a bathroom, a small fridge, TV and video games in my room. My husband (Thank God for this man) prepared all my meals. Whenever I needed something, I would call him on my cell phone. I think a "bell" would've annoyed him ... lol!

I was diagnosed with COVID-19 on July 4th. For the next week, I tried combating my body aches, fever and blood tinged mucous with more Aleve, Advil, Nyquil & Mucinex but NOTHING subsided my symptoms. By Sunday, July 12th, this was the tide that turned the table. It was hard to walk & breathe at the same time. Using my oxygen oximeter (O_2 oximeter), which detects the level or saturation of oxygen in the blood by putting a probe on your finger. My O_2 Sat. was 86%-88% (normal range 95%-100%). I breathlessly told my husband to get a O_2 tank & nasal cannula (my mom's stash) from the closet downstairs.

Once I attached the tubing to the O_2 tank, I put the cannula on and turned the O_2 on to 2 liters but after fifteen to thirty minutes, my O_2 Sat. would not rise above 86%. I decided at that time to pack a bag and head to the ER on base because I didn't want my oxygen saturation to drop so low that I would have to be put on a ventilator.

When we got to the ER, the doctors thought I was a COPD (chronic obstructive pulmonary disease) patient because I had the oxygen, the O_2 oximeter on my finger and looking like I was at death's door. In the ER, I was given a CT scan, which revealed I had 50% bilateral lung capacity or double pneumonia brought on by the coronavirus. I was immediately admitted to the ICU, where I was given a five-day regimen of;

- Remdesivir IV (pronounced Rim*dis*sir*veer) five-to-ten-day trial drug for the COVID-19, that hasn't been approved by the FDA

- Dexamethasone (pronounced Dex*ah*meth*ah*zone) a steroid to treat the inflammation in the lungs
- Rocephin IV (pronounced Ro*ce*fin) antibiotic used to treat bacterial infections.
- Protonix (pronounced Pro*ton*iks) used to treat acid reflux and a persistent cough.
- I also had to have my blood sugars monitored due to the Dexamethasone, which spiked my levels. If my blood sugars were above 150, I was covered with Novolog insulin and for the record I'm not a diabetic!

Once I became stable & the coronavirus started to dissipate, I was released from the hospital on July 17th. I went home & self-quarantined for a week. Went and got retested on July 26th and received my negative results on July 28th.

The coronavirus has taught me life is short & precious! I cherish each and every person that touched my life during this ordeal. COVID-19 has rendered me to the aftereffects of brain fog, some shortness of breath, numbness in my feet, and joint pain. Moving forward, I want to partake in everything and anything but jumping out a plane!!

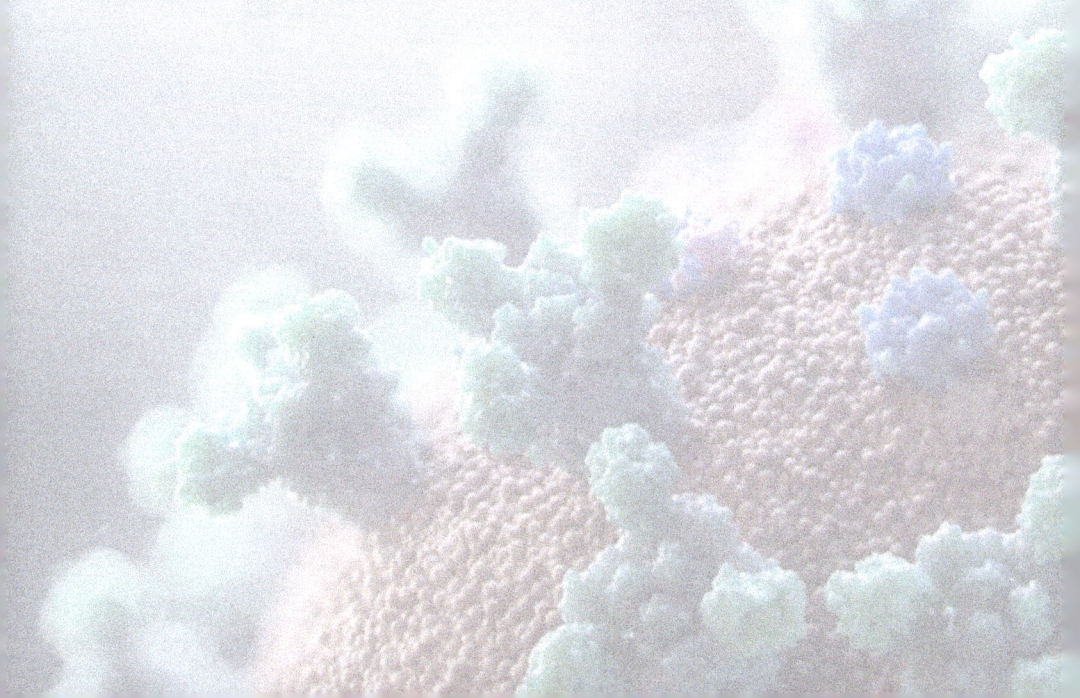

MY NEW NORMAL

Curtis Motley

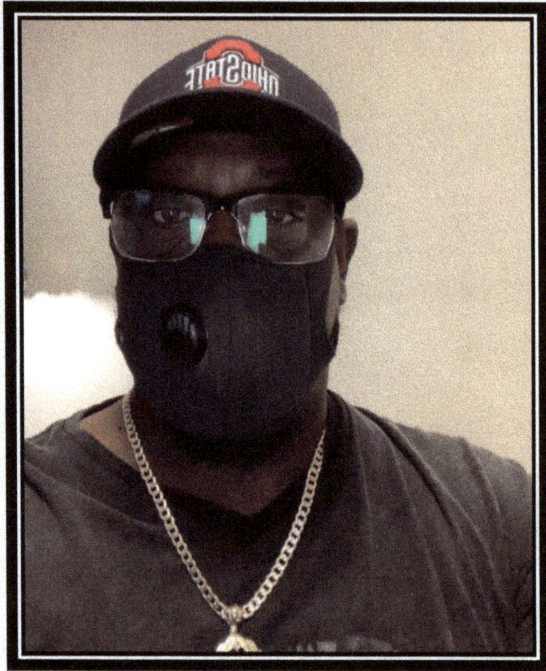

I caught COVID sometime in July 2020. I cannot pinpoint the day, but I started feeling weird: I had a head cold; my sinuses were stopped up; and I had an extreme pain from my head. So, I went out and brought a lot of cold medicine and started dosing up to shake this cold. I started getting body aches and chills. I am on dialysis, and I need a kidney, so when I went on my regular routine to dialysis, I could not take it because I had bad chills and was shaking badly. The technician took me off the machine and let me know that I had to go to the hospital to get checked. I went to the ER room; I was diagnosed with COVID.

I was high risk because I have diabetes and on dialysis. I was admitted into the Orange Park Hospital, and my situation had gotten worse. I was put on oxygen because I had problems breathing, and I did not have an appetite. There was very little that they could do for me since there has not been a specific medicine for COVID, and I was not feeling any better either. My body was weak, but I was not in much pain, I just did not like the oxygen tubes in my nose; it was very uncomfortable. I did get the plasma while I was in the hospital, and it did make me feel better!

After my 11th day in the hospital, I was feeling better but weak. I was in a room with another patient that was COVID-positive also, and he was irate and rude to the nurses. He also had a problem yelling through the night, so I asked for another room. They could not accommodate me, so I checked myself out and went home to homecare for which I had a nurse coming by two days a week to make sure my oxygen was good and to check vitals. Once I went home, I was still in quarantine, and this COVID affected my wife also by her having to also quarantine for three weeks because her job is in the health field. She was also tested before they let her come back to work, and it was negative.

My wife took very good care of me once I got home. I had hot ginger tea every morning, and she made sure I was comfortable. She had to sleep downstairs on an air mattress, so her sacrifice was amazing. What got me through this was my faith in God and all of the prayers I received from family and friends. I had to go to a COVID dialysis center until I tested negative twice. I was still weak after my negative test, so I stayed home for another two weeks, and then I went back to work. My advice is to take this COVID-19 seriously! Wear your mask, wash your hands, and social distance because this may become the new normal.

A Tribute to my Daddy, Willie H. Hampton

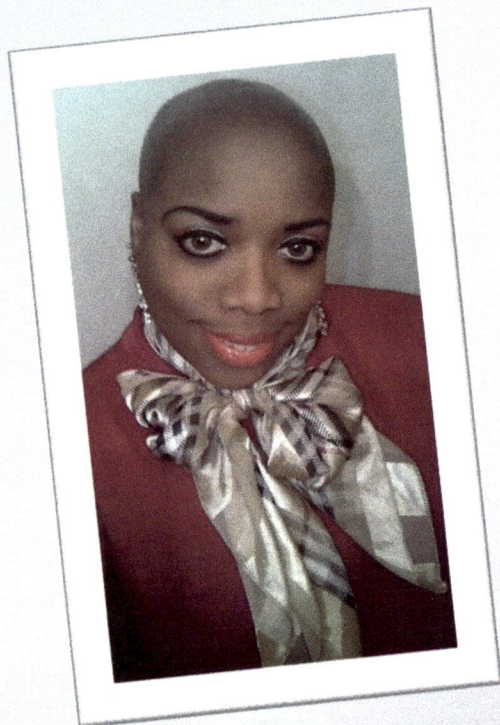

T hursday April 16, 2020, will be a date I will never forget. That was the day I lost my father from COVID-19.

My father was a strong and distinguished man that did not take any mess from anyone. He had underlying illnesses such as diabetes and high blood pressure which had been controlled for several years. On March 27th, I received a call from my mom stating my father had to be rushed to the hospital. The paramedics informed my mom there were no available beds or rooms at the hospital in Albany, Georgia. My father had to be transferred to Macon Memorial Hospital in Macon, Georgia. Once there, he was given a coronavirus test, was diagnosed with COVID-19, and placed on a ventilator machine. On April 16, 2020, my father Willie H. Hampton passed away from COVID-19.

Willie H. Hampton, 73, was from Albany, Georgia. He was born in 1946 in Donalsonville, Georgia, to the late Howard and Ola V. Hampton, both of Seminole County, Georgia.

My father was a loving husband to my mother Mary Hampton for 39 years, and the stepfather to me and my two brothers, William Newbill Jr. and Marlo Newbill Sr.

He will truly be missed but will never be forgotten.

Love you, R.I.P. Daddy

In Loving Memory of

Willie H. Hampton

19th October, 1946 to 16th April, 2020

Willie H. Hampton

Mr. Hampton, 73, was from Albany, GA. He was born in 1946 in Donalsonville, GA to the late Howard and Ola V. Hampton, both of Seminole County, GA.

He was a loving husband to Mary Hampton for 39 years. He is the stepfather to William Newbill, Jr., Tracy Etheridge, and Marlo Newbill Sr.

He will truly be missed but he will never be forgotten.

Love you, R.I.P. Daddy

IT HAPPENED IN A MOMENT

Chaconna Downs

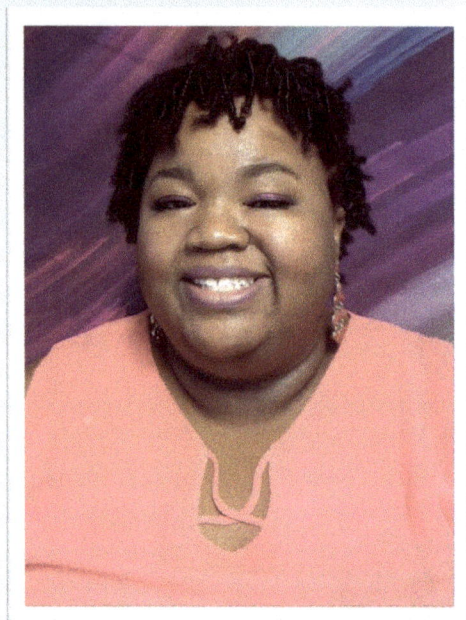

What happens in a moment can change your life forever. I was sitting on my couch when I received a phone call from a close friend saying his daughter's mother was in the hospital with COVID-19, and he needed help caring for her. When he brought the baby to me and told me what was going on, God spoke immediately and told me that the baby's mother wasn't coming home. That's not the kind of thing you share with the father of an 18-month-old baby who's never been a single parent. I fasted and prayed that God would bless her mother to be healed on this side, but deep down I knew what He said wouldn't change.

In the days to come, I would get up extra early to make sure things were prepared for her and wait to see her little face each morning. Every morning, she would greet me with those big bright eyes and the sweetest little smile. All the while her mom was fighting for her life and her big brother was three hours away wondering when mommy would be home. God has a funny way of orchestrating things to work together for our good.

I was already working primarily from home, and my boss was extremely understanding. My coworkers, friends, family, and even strangers rallied to help my sweet little baby. God blessed her with everything she needed during the most transitional time of her little life. She had no idea that her mom was about to transition home to be with the Father, and neither did her dad. I did what I could to help him get prepared without telling him what God had spoken, but there's really nothing that prepares you to lose a loved one, let alone the mother of your child.

The day her mother transitioned, she was here with me, and her dad walked in a little after noon. I lifted my head to see a stunned look on his face, tear-stained cheeks, and hear the choked back words, "She's gone." I was finishing up a virtual therapy appointment with a client and quickly had to shift gears. He grabbed his daughter, held her tight, and then clutched his head in disbelief. I ended my session, went to him, and held him for a few minutes to reassure him that he wasn't alone. I had peace and was somehow prepared for that moment even though I'd wished a thousand times it wouldn't have to come so soon.

After that, her dad had a lot of sleepless nights and big feelings he didn't quite know how to handle. I did what I do best: pray! I called on my friends and family to cover them in prayer; I prayed with him when he was here and covered the baby whenever she was with me. We quickly settled into a routine and began to establish a sense of normal for her. She had her toys and her favorite blanket that doubled as a booster seat, her baby doll that my mom was so adamant about me getting for her, and her spot on the couch.

To look into her eyes, you would never know we're in the middle of a pandemic, and that loved ones are dying all around us. All I saw was innocence, joy, hope, peace, and unconditional love. We showered each other with love, hugs, and kisses. She fed me cheerios and laughed when I would pretend to eat her fingers.

She would wake up singing, and I would hear Jesus . . . Jesus . . . Jesus . . . in her little broken baby tone coming sweetly from my room.   Her giggles filled my home and heart with joy unspeakable. I don't know God's plan, but I surely do appreciate Him painting me into her picture. Although my stinky baby is leaving me in a few short days, I rest assured knowing that she has a strong village, a group of mothers who love her both near and far, and a lot of new family that will keep her lifted in prayer. She has something great and mighty to do in this earth realm, and even if it was only but for a moment, I got to love her.

**And now, for our final contribution to this volume
and to this series...**

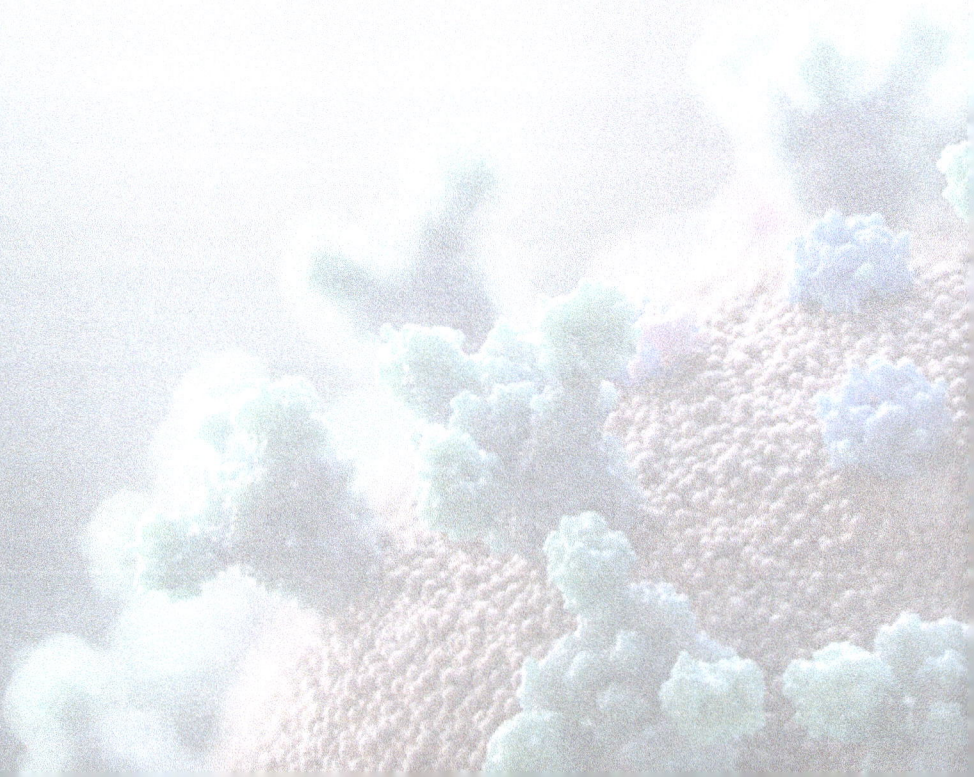

AUTHOR CHAD "BRANDON" BUTLER

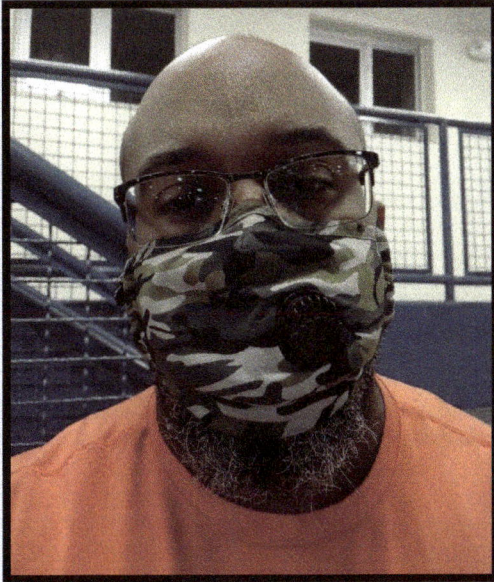

My name is Chad Butler, and I recently turned forty years old. I am a serial entrepreneur, enjoy learning about technology, and in the early months of the pandemic of 2020, I was diagnosed with COVID-19.

When were you experiencing symptoms from the COVID-19 Virus?

It was around March 23, 2020, that I knew there was something wrong. I went to the doctor to get an x-ray to rule out COVID, actually. I had the flu in the beginning parts of the month, and I was COVID-19 negative during that time. I had similar symptoms, and I told myself, "Okay, I'm going to go to the doctor so they can say, "Hey, it's the flu again. You don't have COVID", and I figured they would give me a routine chest x-ray and another prescription, but when I got there, they said, "No, you have it."

It's my understanding that you don't particularly enjoy going to the doctor. What prompted you to go to the doctor a second time in the same month?

I had an off and on fever, and I was super tired. I was more lethargic than usual; work was the only time my adrenaline kept me going. My body was extremely tired.

Did you try to self-medicate?

I doped up every day with over-the-counter medication.

So, when you went to the doctor earlier in March, they didn't prescribe anything?

They prescribed an Albuterol inhaler which I never picked up from the pharmacy. Of course, now every time I go to any doctor's appointment, they mention it, and I merely point out that I'm not taking Albuterol. I am not asthmatic at this time and never have been.

Why didn't you take the Albuterol?

I didn't need it; I wasn't having trouble breathing. I don't know why it was prescribed in the first place. Western doctors like to throw medicine on people. I never indicated any discomfort or trouble with breathing; I didn't have any lung problems.

What type of at-home remedies did you attempt to try and feel better?

I drank fluids, tried to rest and ... life goes on.

You said that you were lethargic. I know that your daily work is quite physical; how did you combat that tiredness?

It didn't bother me while I was at work, but when I would get home, I would shower, lie down, and sleep for three to four hours which is unlike me.

Did you have a daily fever?

I didn't check myself daily, but when I did check, there was an up and down fever. It didn't leave until I was in the hospital for two days without one.

Please tell me how the hospital stay came about.

I went to get the x-ray so they could tell me it's just the flu again. They ran a test and had me sit in a negative-pressure room (a room that doesn't allow air to circulate so when you're breathing it all funnels toward an air machine like a suction) for two hours while they waited for the results. They initially did an x-ray which confirmed that I had pneumonia. They drew blood which confirmed that I had the flu and also confirmed that I had COVID-19.

What were you thinking?

That I just wanted to go home. There was no TV; the battery on my phone was about to die from social-media trolling for two hours. This was at one local hospital where I went for the routine x-ray. Once it was determined that I indeed had COVID-19, I was whisked away in an ambulance to another hospital.

What was that like? What was your first thought when they told you that you were positive for COVID-19?

I was shocked and in disbelief because I didn't have any of the symptoms that were reported nationally and internationally until I actually thought about it. The fever was extensive, but they didn't know that the fatigue was a symptom. I never coughed, and I didn't feel sick; it was so early on that they didn't include fatigue as a symptom.

Were you admitted into a private room?

Yes.

Have you ever stayed in the hospital before?

No.

What type of medication did they give you while you were in the hospital?

The first two days I had an IV, and they were giving me Hydroxychloroquine which is an immunosuppressive. At the time, it was supposed to be a wonder drug since it was known to be a "cure" for COVID-19. It has since been determined that it does not heal an individual from the virus.

Were you able to get in touch with your family?

Yes, when I had my diagnosis, but at that point, I had to sit and wait, which was before I went to the second hospital.

How long were you in the hospital?

Too long, in my opinion: eight to ten days almost.

What type of issues did you have in the hospital as you were experiencing the virus?

The fever was sporadic, and I had diarrhea. I never had diarrhea before I was admitted; it was surely COVID-19-related, and it was an indescribable smell that I'll never forget.

Sometimes COVID-19 is a death sentence in people's minds. Were you ever worried that you wouldn't make it out of the hospital?

No. By the time I was admitted, I was feeling bad, but I didn't feel like death like some people describe. Was it scary that this could have been my fate? Yes, but did I think I was going to die? No.

In speaking to other COVID-19 survivors, your story seems incredible. Do you feel that your memory was affected at all?

No.

Since your diagnosis and ultimately, your healing, what type of experiences have you had from professionals related to the disease?

Well, while I was in the hospital, I involuntarily donated many vials of blood (I gather it was for research for a cure since I recovered from my three consecutive illnesses so fast.) I had different interviews with different counties' health departments. Everyone seemed to not believe I was not experiencing the same, extraordinary symptoms and fatalities that were happening around me.

I know you have a large family. How was your post-hospital time at home?

I came home and rested for a few days and then went back to work. As a slight precaution, I separated myself from my family and the house had already been disinfected.

What was recommended for you? A self-quarantine of at least two weeks?

No, because I was already in the hospital for a week, and my contagious stage ended two days after I left the hospital. I didn't have to worry about contagion, but they said I would be really, really tired upon leaving, and I was. I lost thirty-five pounds, and I didn't realize just how diminished my stamina was. Other than that, I didn't have to do any quarantine or anything like that.

And none of your family was affected during your contagious period when you thought you had the flu?

No. I'm the only person that contracted the plague, thankfully.

How do you think you contracted COVID-19?

I don't speculate, because it doesn't really matter. I do have suspicion, however. Due to contact from an attorney, I may have contracted this disease from an acquaintance I met for business purposes in a night club. The club housed many infected individuals and was ultimately closed and has not re-opened.

Do you have any repercussions, any PTSD symptoms?

Yes, I have PTSD. I wear my mask religiously; however, I don't segregate from anything that I want or need to do. I breathe differently because I ate through my feelings, and I've gained forty pounds in three months.

I know you're a pretty introverted person, and I thank you for chatting with me. Your story will encourage others. What made you decide to share?

Intense, immense pressure from external sources. LOL. My dear friend asked me to share this story and, though it is still very fresh in my life, I decided I would.

Do you have any encouraging words for others?

Yes: don't be afraid to live. Sitting in a hospital room not knowing what's next gives a unique perspective on "living" as opposed to being afraid to die. My words to share would be, "Don't be afraid to live."

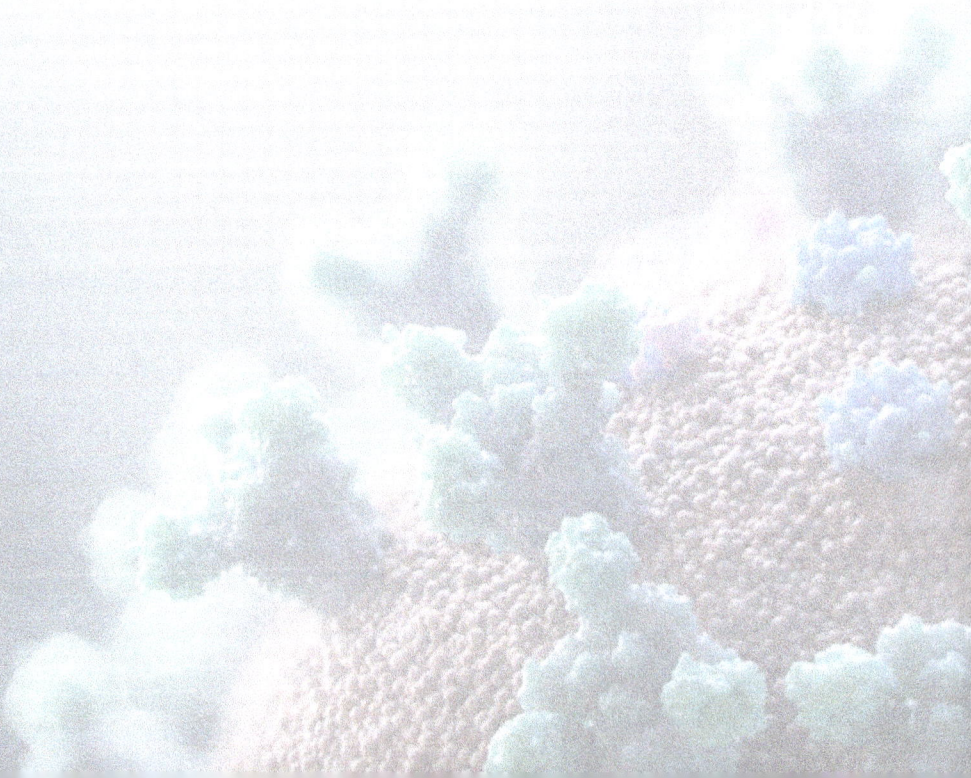

This concludes *Confinement Chronicles*, **Even in My Darkest Hour - You Never Left Me.**

As we now end Volume X, we encourage you to order the first nine volumes and follow *Confinement Chronicles* by Angie BEE Productions on Facebook. As we now prepare to travel and meet each of you in various locations throughout the United States beginning in 2021, we pray that you share what you have learned with others, and join with us to lead them to a relationship with Christ.

Again, thank you to Theresa Jordan of *Triumphant Magazine* and Donna Gray-Banks of the F.R.E.S.H. Book Festival for serving as our promotional sponsors during this series. Thank you to my precious sister Sonya Bennett who served as narrator in several volumes. Special thanks to the members of our evangelism troupe for praying for me, writing for us, and for making plans to join us on during the tour.

I would also like to thank my family for encouraging me to complete this project, especially my husband Bartee. He cooked, cleaned, cared for me while I healed from surgery, and he loved on me during the production of the *Confinement Chronicles* series, and for this alone ... I will ALWAYS be grateful. Thank you, Jesus!

BEE Blessed

Sincerely,

Evangelist Angie BEE

THE AUTHORS

In Order of Appearance

Penekala "Neka" Perkins is a Senior Labor Relations Advisor with the Department of the Navy and an author. She is also the owner of Kids Need Faith 2, LLC and Momager of her six-year-old daughter, Faith.

Follow her online via Facebook: www.facebook.com/AuthorNekaPerkins or send an email to Nekatheauthor@gmail.com.

Sonya Bennett, a native Detroiter, has worn many titles in her 49 years of existence: Daughter, Sister, Aunt, Mother, Community Advocate and, most recently: Author. A former court stenographer that holds an English Degree: Ms. Bennett's love of words began in elementary school when spelling bee terms became inspiration for definition-diving the old-fashioned way: in a dictionary. From understanding came compilation: poems. From poems came public speaking and, as they say, the rest is HERstory.

Laughter, bluntness and honesty surround the lines of Ms. Bennett's stories that are based loosely (and not so loosely) on her life. Names have been changed and scenarios altered; however, as she quips often: the TRUTH never changes.

Ever evolving, always creating, striving for that moment when I read, "Local Girl Does Well", Ms. Bennett's favorite scripture is Philippians 4:13.

Follow her online at www.Facebook.com/AuthorSonyaBennett

Monique Chandler is a Distinguished International Toastmaster, Consultant, Educator and Author of the book *Reconnecting with Your Happy*. She possesses unique blends of contagious, high volume, motivational energy, and a sincere heart for helping others reach their pinnacle. <u>Visit her online at</u> <u>www.reconnectingwithyourhappy.com</u> and secure a copy of her book: *Reconnecting with Your Happy* on Amazon | Kindle.

Consultant, Educator and Author of "**Hurt People, Help People**". Monique Chandler is a Distinguished International Toastmaster. She possesses a unique blend of contagious, high volume, motivational energy, and a sincere heart for helping others reach their pinnacle.

Don't delay, purchase your order today!
www.reconnectingwithyourhappy.com
CashApp: $beconnected
Additional published books:
Reconnecting With Your Happy
Finding Joy In The Journey, International Best Seller
Confinement Chronicles, Volume I – "The Game Changer"
& Volume IV – "Hurt People, Help People"
Monique A. Chandler, MBA, DTM
Author | Consultant | Educator |

Rue Mayweather is a former adjunct professor and the author of the *Memoir, No Gold at the End of the Rainbow.* With more than a decade of writing Reso-ology (Resolutions plus Biographies) for fallen military and law enforcement officers and their families, Rue has a unique way of blending a story to capture an audience, thus bringing sunshine to the bleakest situations.

Rue earned her M.S.E. from Amberton University, and is a certified Red Team analyst and a military veteran. She LOVES succulent plants, especially if they're rare.
Recipe for a Man (She Thought) is Rue's second book.

Rue Mayweather is an Authorpreneur and lives in Dallas, Texas. Rue help others re-birth their forgotten gifts of "RUE (Rare, Unique and Essential) by changing first assisting in changing their attitude; then showing how to employ

RUE to branch multiple streams of income. Visit www.ruemayweather.com or send an email to rmayweather@prodigy.net

Terri B. Jones Live is a company that makes publishing your Alexa Skills content on Amazon Echo devices easy. Terri has published 16 Alexa Skills on Amazon Alexa Echo devices. With the help of Alexa Skills Expert, Terri Jones, you will create an Alexa Skill you can get up and running in as little time as 48 hours! Probably the hardest part is deciding which Alexa Skill you want to make first.

As the founder of Terri B. Jones Live, she is a highly sought-after Speaker, Author, Trainer, Coach, Course Creator, Website Designer, Online Marketer, Amazon Skills and Google Actions Developer. Terri, graduated from Phillips University in 1984 with a degree in Computer Programming and University of Phoenix Jacksonville, FL location in 2003 with a degree in Business Information Systems. Terri has worked in IT for over 33 years. She is the Marketing Strategies Admin in the Black Owned Business Jacksonville Facebook Group with over 6k members. In (BOBSJax) she teaches weekly marketing strategies to keep local businesses abreast of online marketing strategies to grow brand, reach and revenue and retirement readiness strategies.

https://terribjones.com/voiceintegration
https://wevoiceit.com
https://youtube.com/terrijones
https://facebook.com/terribjoneslive

Vernessa Blackwell is an author, and certified grief support and joy restoration coach. The loss of both parents and all her siblings, to include three sisters and a brother, sparked her purposeful journey into coaching. Vernessa is the author of The Grief Helpline. Additionally, she is a mentor, expo host, and speaker. She is known as "The Grief Strategist". Dedicated to inspiring and empowering individuals for personal and professional success, Vernessa Blackwell is known for challenging and motivating clients to take action and move forward in grief and life transitions. She is a passionate, energetic, and charming presenter who engages her audience with inspiring, interactive workshops. She specialized in Joy Restoration Coaching. Vernessa has a heart for serving and wants to see people healed and set free. She has received her healing from the Lord. She understands what you are going through and knows how to get you through it.

Through coaching, training, and mentoring, Vernessa Blackwell offers hope, encouragement, and support as individuals navigate the challenges and adversities of life and loss. She is the founder of the Grief Helpline. She conducts presentations, offers workshops, in-service training, assemblies, classroom programs and keynotes on topics pertaining to grief in the lives of children, teens and adults faced with different types of loss. Vernessa Blackwell serves as a grief consultant and grief counselor for teenagers, adults, families, groups and for communities following a loss of any type. Vernessa has an office in Southern Maryland. She provides sessionsvia Skype and by phone, and also makes home visits or community calls as a consultant. She conducts presentations and training programs throughout the U.S. and Canada. You can Vernessa Blackwell on fb Instagram and linked in as the Grief Strategist.

Evangelist Tahara Lee

- Born in Easton, Maryland
- Oldest child of five – 2 girls, three boys
- Baptized at age 12 in Silver Lake, Dover, Delaware / Receiver of the Holy Spirit
- Mother of four daughters / Grandmother of 11 – 4 girls (one deceased), 7 boys

- Moved to Orlando, Florida, in 1993
- Macedonia Missionary Baptist Church, Community Baptist Church, Life Focus Ministries, Divine Orders International Ministries
- Baptized/Rededication at age 37 at Community Baptist Church. Positions; taught women's Sunday School, taught children's Wednesday night bible study. Released from Community Baptist in good standing
- Life Focus Ministries – Winter Garden, Florida. Positions; Usher, Finance Officer, Evangelistic Team, Intercessor Prayer Warrior. Released from Life Focus Ministry in good standing
- Helped birth vision • Divine Orders International Ministry. After 3 years of service ordained Evangelist by Board of Bishops of covering church • Love Center Ministries, Apalachicola, Florida, Apostle Shirley C. White, Overseer
- Birthed Alabaster Box Ministry. Intercessory Prayer Warrior. Confidant for Christ (confidential meetings). Praise Dancer. Flag Ministry
- Serves as a Ministry Leader of *The Tour That Angie BEE Presents* 2012 to Present.
- Traveling Evangelist, Ministers, Authors, Poets, Singers, Praise Dancers, Entrepreneurs, Videographers.
- I seek God with my whole heart. An obedient servant to the Lord, Abba Father.

Thaddeus Randolph is a Bronze Star recipient and retired U.S. Army veteran of 21 years. He has a Bachelor of Science in Business Administration from Strayer University and a Master of Arts in Pastoral Counseling from Liberty University. Thaddeus currently Serves as Ministries Director at Strong Tower Church in Fredericksburg, Virginia. He and his wife Amanda (also a retired Army Veteran) reside in Fredericksburg, VA with their two sons, Samuel and Xavier. Social Media Contact: totalgracesolutions@gmail.com
thadd88@gmail.com
totalgracesolutions.com

www.facebook.com/thadd88
www.facebook.com/thadandamana www.instagram.com/randolphthads

Bartee is affectionately referred to as "The Rage of The Stage" here in Central Florida. This sensational R&B singer began his career at the age of eleven in his hometown of Akron, Ohio. He continues to share his natural-born feeling for music just as aggressively as he first did decades ago. Always sought after, Bartee is a versatile entertainer that performs Smooth Jazz, Vintage Soul, and a beautiful Motown Review.

Bartee has shared the stage with music icons such as James Ingram, Howard Hewitt, The Ohio Players, Linda Cole, and The O'Jays. Bartee leads the Dads-on-Duty workshop while on *The TOUR that Angie BEE Presents*, and he leads by Angie BEE's side in the God, Me & You Workshop, as well. You can find Bartee performing a Motown Review concert during the TOUR weekend retreats for couples, and he continues to serve the Lord with gladness through his lifestyle and commitment to his family.

In 2013, Bartee met, dated, and married Angie BEE in less than six months. Before he met her, he vowed to NEVER remarry, and she vowed NEVER to submit to another man. God orchestrated something different for the two of them, and their book reveals the details.

Bartee first became a published author on August 1, 2017. As co-author, he and his wife Angie BEE wrote *In the Beginning: There Was God, Me & You*, published by Ladero Press. This book reveals their true love story that only God could have written. Bartee always wanted to write a book and he will soon write his life story of juvenile incarceration to prison, and God's many blessings in his life.

Together, Bartee and Angie BEE have two sons, two daughters and two brand new sons-in-law. Search for Bartee online at www.BarteeSings.com and follow him on search for at www.facebook.com/pg/BarteeTheAuthor

You know, my husband may joke around a bit about my round, bald head, but he is truthful about ONE thing...most men (people) can recognize a person wearing a wig from a mile away! Why do we wear them? Are we trying to impress somebody else or do we cover our heads in shame? Either way, I appreciate my husband's jovial nature about my bald head. Even though he is bald-by-choice, I appreciate HIS bald head, too!

Regina Nunnally is a native of Daytona Beach, Florida. She is a criminal defense attorney, ordained minister, and associate pastor at Restoration Church. Regina is a travelista entrepreneur and contributing author to an Amazon.com best seller "Dailey Dose Women in Business." Loving to express herself, Regina hosts a weekly Tuesday night online event called "See The World Thru My Eyes" and has written numerous articles for both online and offline publications. Every Friday she posts inspirational lipsync videos on various social media outlets. She loves to travel, collards greens and garlic crabs.

Christopher M. Swansburg, 31, served six years in the Army, and is a Veteran of Afghanistan. He holds a Bachelor's degree in business management and served as in intern with Angie BEE Productions for the past three years. He currently works as an automotive technician, and he loves working with wood. Swansburg has an interest in exotic pets. He and his bride wed on October 31, 2020.

Ivy Sebastien was born Nov 28th, 1975 in Brooklyn New York. She is a Dancer, Writer, Entrepreneur, Motivational Speaker and Life Coach; she also carries a BS in Criminal l Justice and minor in Human Service / Counseling. A licensed Minister, Ivy has worked with inner city youth and young adults in counseling in drugs and rehabilitation and Dance, she loves to do outreach and work with the community to make a change.

Marcus Latimer is a Retired Letter Carrier after serving for 34 years in Detroit, Michigan.

He enjoys serving his community through the Detroit Westown Hartford Lions Club and the Thomara Latimer Cancer Foundation.

He is a life-long member of Hartford Memorial Baptist Church in Detroit Michigan having served on the Young Adult Choir, the Cathedral Choir, the Jubilee Chorus & the Male Chorus. Latimer is also a member of the Trustee Board.

The Thomara Latimer Cancer Foundation gives $1,000.00 scholarships to patients. They coordinate resources with respect to cause, prevention, treatment and care of pediatric and young adult cancer patients. Some examples are transportation for appointments, medication and other needs. Latimer supports the membership and fundraising efforts www.Thomlatimercares.org.

You may contact Marcus Latimer via email at: mlfree@kateibo.com

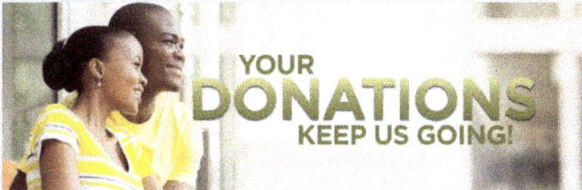

Dr. April L. (Henderson) Johnson, was born and raised in Manchester, New Jersey. In 2004, she moved to Florida where she currently resides with her husband, Samuel Johnson. Dr. Johnson has four sons: Jarron, Jay, Mark and Justin. She is a proud grandmother of six grandchildren.

Dr. A.J. (as she is affectionately known) earned her Bachelor of Science degree in Political Science from Wesley College, Dover, Delaware in 1995. She went on to receive a master's degree in Biblical Studies at Calvary Bible Institute, Dover, Delaware. In August 2019, she earned her doctoral degree in Christian Counseling from Friends International Christian University.

Dr. April L. Johnson is the Senior Pastor of Saint Mary FreeWill Baptist Church, 410 Hunter Street, Plant City, Florida.

Currently, Dr. Johnson is employed as a Vice President and Senior Manager of a financial center at one of the country's largest banks. Additionally, she serves as a member on the Board of Directors, Pregnancy Care Center Non-Profit Organization in Plant City, Florida

Her heart is to be an effective leader & builder of community relationships through outreach with an emphasis in financial & literacy programs.

With maintaining a positive area of influence, she works with many organizations within the community and online to help others become strong spiritually, mentally and financially.

Tamara Mackroy has collectively over twenty years of experience in supervising programs, managing compliance regulations, and overseeing payer contracts. Tamara has worked as a NY State Certified Physical Therapy Aide, has her AAS as a Medical Assistant, her BBA in Health Services Administration and has her MS in Human Services with a Concentration in Social Policy, Analysis and Planning. She is certified in Project Management Essentials and is Lean Six Sigma Yellow Belt certified. She has sat on a few Central Florida boards and is a member of many organizations. In her role as Project Management Consultant, she works with Human Services providers in helping them strengthen business operations to further push their organizational missions in being able to help those living in our communities.

Tamara Mackroy, M.S.H.S., PMEC, Lean 6σ Certified
Owner/Project Management Consultant
Management & Consultative Favor, LLC (MaCFavor)
407-436-7825
macfavor.com

With the **FAVOR** *of God over your life, all things are possible...*

Karen Chandler is as an Associate Pastor and Prayer Leader and uses insight attained in the trenches of life to answer questions that people of faith want to ask. Karen is that trusted friend, that will listen without judging. She is also known for giving wise advice. Karen lives Jarrell, Texas and can be reached on Facebook and you can also reach her by sending an email to sisinthespirit@gmail.com

Althea Ross Chavers, who simply calls herself The Beautiful Althea, is the First Lady of the St. James Missionary Baptist Church in the city of Osteen, FL is married to Pastor Larry D. Chavers, Sr. At the time of this printing, the two have celebrated thirty-two years of marriage, and through this union, they have four beautiful children. She is a grandma of two and the godmother of thirty (30!) children.

The Beautiful Althea has dedicated her life to service; she finds joy in serving the youth of her church and the youth of her community.

She has mentored and nurtured youth ages six to eighteen, at the Lacey Family/Spring Hill Boys & Girls Club for nineteen years, and before that, she mentored kids ages two to six years old at the Twinkle Star Montessori School for seventeen years. First Lady Chavers feels it as an honor to be able to serve in the community where she was born and raised with her other sisters and brothers.

The Beautiful Althea sits on many boards throughout her community she has received numerous awards in her lifetime, but it must mentioned: the Clarence "Bo" Davenport, Community Legacy Recognition, Straight Outta Spring Hill Torch of Hope Award given to her by the Westside Martin Luther King Jr. Committee in the honor of a man that she truly looks up to. The Beautiful Althea is featured on the mural in her community, and although grateful for it all, she realizes that it does not make her the person she is today; it's the standards and moral values that were instilled in me from her mom Mrs. Katie Lee Singleton. "Mom made sure we were respectful to others with no questions asked."

The Beautiful Althea often tells people, "If you don't know love, you don't know me. If you need love, here I am." Then, she is ready to give you a hug.

The Beautiful Althea's favorite scripture is Philippians 4:13, *I can do all things through Christ who strengthen me.*

Favorite motto: If I can help somebody as I pass along the way, then my living will not be in vain.

Althea Ross Chavers, a wife, a mother, a First Lady, an Evangelist, a teacher, a mentor, a 10-year breast cancer survivor, and yes, a Bethune Cookman Wildcat, but most of all a servant to God's people.

Reverend Dawn Martin is an Associate Minister at Omega Baptist Church where she serves under the leadership of Pastor Daryl Ward and Co- Pastor Vanessa Oliver Ward. Dawn has received her BA in Human Services, and a Masters in Human Service and is currently working on a PHD in Human Services with a focus on community and family. Reverend Martin currently is the founder of Just Dazzlind Productions, Diva By Design Ministries, and Girl Empowered and Mentored to Success (G.E.M.S) which is a complete Educational and Success tool for women, girls and teenaged young ladies. Her plan is to develop long lasting partnerships to help create a better world. Her goal is to uplift, enhance, motivate, and celebrate women and girls.

Dawn is pleased to say that the public has fully embraced her purpose and has opened its doors for more information. The newly published author of Fill My Cup-Transitioning to your Purpose, My Morning Cup (Women's Journal) and My Cup Is Half Full (Teen Girls Journal), I Am (Journal to Positive Speaking), and Creating the Man (Teen Boys Journal). Dawn continues to share her life's journey, personally and professionally, as she helps others recognize their life's purpose.

Dawn Martin hopes that all will join her in the development, enhancement, motivation and education of those building success.

Accomplishments:

G.E.M.S- Girls Motivated and Mentored to Success
G.E.N.T.S- Gentlemen Encouraged and Nurtured to Success
Divas By Design Radio & TV Host
Divas Stomp The Runway- Choreographer & Promoter
Women On Assignment Conference- Facilitator
My Morning Cup- Journal for Women.

For further information or to request a speaking engagement: Rev. Dawn Martin
Dazzlind2001@yahoo.com www.blogtalkradio.com/Dazzlind
937-270-8118

Rex al Opusunju, D.Div, is the Presiding Bishop, Abounding Love Christian Centre Nigeria. He was born September 19, 1967, in Umuahia Abia State, Nigeria. He is Bible teacher, researcher, inspired Christian author, and conference/motivational speaker. He is a Marquis Who's Who Listee- (Marquis Who's Who in the World 26th Edition 2009). He is married to Believe Mlumun Akudo Opusunju (March 23, 1996) and lives in Umuahia, Abia State, Nigeria.

Ronald Stafford is a handsome, well-blessed, respectful and calm Jacksonville resident that looks forward to turning 40 in 2021. Both sides of his praying family are big! Stafford has no children and he is constantly writing.

Ronald has spent nearly seven years in various prisons. While serving his time in prison, he started to get his thoughts together, and when he got out of prison five years ago, he began to write his first book.

In October of 2020, Stafford was introduced to Angie BEE Productions. This agency was tasked to produce his book as an audiobook. He even contributed to the inspirational audiobook compilation series titled *Confinement Chronicles*.

Ronald believes that it is important for him to keep writing and promote his writings because: "A lot of ears need to hear, and my writings should help others in life to not make the same mistakes that I made."

Contact the author at 904-862-9948 or via email at Ronaldlamont38@gmail.com

Pastor Patrick Wilkerson was born in Enterprise, Alabama, the oldest of five siblings. He attended the local schools there where he was active in the local church and community. He moved to Daytona Beach, Florida, where he currently resides, and met his wife of twenty-two years, Karen Wilkerson, and has one daughter, Patrice Wilkerson. He was called to pastor the St. James Missionary Baptist Church of Bunnell, Florida, in May of 2005, and has served and led faithfully for twelve years.

Pastor Wilkerson's professional career includes Shift Supervisor with the State of Florida Department of Juvenile Justice, Program Administrator of First Step Adolescence Services, Director of Volusia Halfway House and Campus Advisor/Athletic Coach with Volusia County School Board, and Huddle Leader for Fellowship of Christian Athletes. He attended Troy State University where he majored in Sociology. He received his Bachelors of Theology in June of 2010, from Progressive Baptist Seminary in Jacksonville, Florida and received his Doctorate of Divinity from St. Thomas Christian University. Wilkerson is the former facilitator for the USJA Congress of Christian Education and a national certified teacher of church history and theology. He is the former President of the Union St. James Association Southern District and former 1st Vice Moderator of Union St. James Association. His life desires are to educate, teach and train Gods' people on a regular basis about their true purpose in society, encourage and motivate them to respect others, and to strive for spiritual excellence.

He encourages the youth spiritually and professionally, to complete their education in order to become productive within our society/community and to live a life that is pleasing to God. Pastor Wilkerson is a mentor to youth of all

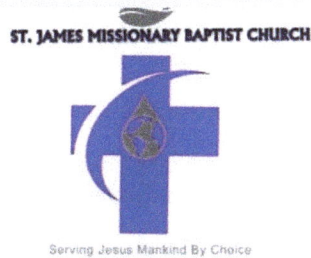

ages and ethnic backgrounds, on a regular basis to identify and correct behavior conflicts. He desires to equip our 'seasoned saints' with knowledge of 21st Century technology to help them embrace the new challenges and changes in life. Pastor Wilkerson endeavors daily to live the life he teaches and preaches to others.

Kami Love is best known for writing books and stories for children, and she does it at the highest level. Kami Love is nine years old and studies in 4th grade. She started writing at the tender age of 7 and was inspired by the writer of her favorite book, Arthur. She decided to choose writing as a profession for herself, and after completing high school, she is going to attend college where she can learn more about writing skills.

Kami Love is full of joy and makes sure she enjoys every moment of her life as she had a dream about it. Her energy came from her mother, who supports her all the time and encourages her to peruse her dreams as she wants.

The little author has so far written only one e-book, paperback, and audio and plans to write more books and e-books. Kami Love's message for her fellow authors is to " Find your way and Follow your DREAMS."

Signed Kami Love
774-326-0652
www.Shopkamilove.com

Jalen Alexander is a 15-year-old, Arts Studies student born and raised in Detroit, MI. Attending a college-prep high school, Jalen possesses many talents including: visual arts, he has mastered several musical instruments and has traveled extensively competing and excelling in the challenging sport of Chess.

Jalen is a son/brother/grandchild/nephew and a doting uncle that displays respect, a great sense of humor and a sincerely nurturing spirit. He now holds the most auspicious title of Author in his inaugural contribution to the Confinement Chronicles series, expressing his thoughts and feelings about living through this pandemic. Jalen enjoys playing card games, video games and thrilling his family with his magic tricks. Contact Jalen at JSpice414@gmail.com

Dion Taylor is originally from Paterson, New Jersey, and he recently moved to Florida. This is Mr. Taylor's first audiobook contribution, and he would like to dedicate it to his late mother, Betty Jean Johnson and his late grandmother, Eloise Wade. Dion is sixteen years old, and he is a junior in high school. Dion is pursuing a degree and career in computer science and electrical engineering. He knows with God all things are possible. Dion recently became the 1st scholarship winner of the My Joy is Power Scholarship sponsored by Pastor Dr. April Johnson's, *My Joy is Power* book.

Sandra "Bee" is an eight-year-old third grader, born in Michigan. She has been an entrepreneur for the past year. She is a baptized member of Beth Eden Missionary Baptist Church and is a trained voice actress narrating audiobooks for Angie BEE BEE Productions. Sandra has been featured in several national commercials as an actress and has even read books to her peers during ministry outreach workshops! Follow her online at www.Facebook.com/SandraBowBoss

Angie Cowan is a computer support analyst and the owner of AGC Designs, a computer support and design company and now a published author. She is a creative, having started playing drums at age six and piano at age seven, and continued both through high school and into college. The technology side of Angie completed and earned a Bachelor's of Arts Degree from Jacksonville University in Computer Information Systems.

While attempting to start a career in Information Technology, that creative side was always inside of her, which allowed her opportunity to co-write a love ballad called "Natural Love" with a couple of friends, and which was eventually recorded by a band she managed at the time. That song was included on an album the band recorded which she co-produced. Angie has also produced two short films with a couple of local filmmakers in the area.

Writing was never a real thought for Angie, although she did dabble with a few unreleased stories over the years. After dealing with two major life-altering health challenges, and with God's grace and mercy on her life, she knew what God did for her had to be shared in some way. When the opportunity presented itself by Angie BEE, there was some initial self-doubt, but God put a word in her heart and said not to let this opportunity pass.

She has two foundational scriptures for her life.   They are:
Be strong and courageous. Do not be afraid or terrified because of them, for the Lord your God goes with you; he will never leave you nor forsake you. Deuteronomy 31:6 NIV

Now to Him who is able to do exceedingly abundantly above all that we ask or think, according to the power that works in us, to Him be glory in the church by Christ Jesus to all generations, forever and ever. Amen. Ephesians 3:20-21 NKJV

Sharlyne Carla Rogers is an award-winning author, inspirational speaker, and professional editor who has served as an intercessor since 2003, edifying the Body of Christ through prayer and exhortation. She has published seven non-fiction books thus far, including and her latest book titled "Fear? NOT!" Sharlyne also utilizes her gifts and talents via Spirit of Excellence Writing & Editing Services, LLC, contributing articles to magazines as well as editing and proofreading various copy for a broad range of writers and organizations nationwide.

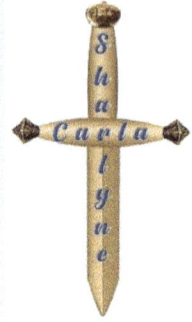

Sharlyne has been invited to speak and teach at a variety of community and ministry events; judged four beauty pageants; and been a guest on several radio and TV shows. Expanding her creativity to stage and screen, she has ministered in dance as well as acted in a Christian hip-hop video, gospel play, short film, commercials, and feature films. Sharlyne also contributed to the script for "The Turnaround" movie, which has won and been nominated for several awards.

Sharlyne holds an MBA in Management and has a Woman & Minority Business Certification from the State of Florida. She has continued to expand her community reach by launching a 501c3 nonprofit charity organization, Sword of the Spirit Ministries Florida, Inc., which was created to empower single parents and their children to become more productive citizens spiritually, physically, and financially. Born and raised in Southern California, Sharlyne currently lives with her husband William in Central Florida.

www.takeupthysword.com

sharlyne@takeupthysword.com

Michelle Walters-Johnson, is the owner of Lady Behind the Wig and the Luxe Hair by Michelle wig line. She's a daughter, a sister, a mother, a wife and a loyal friend. She has a Bachelor's degree in Psychology and a Master's in Business Administration. When she is not slaying wigs or giving advice, she works as an admission counselor helping people accomplish their graduate school dreams.

She suffered from hair loss. Losing her hair caused her to have to seek solutions to camouflage her hair loss, which eventually led her to the world of wigs, which then led her to wanting to share her craft with others. By coming forward with her truth, she believes that she has found her profound purpose and unique ministry.

In the hair business self-esteem is a primary focus. Women especially, base their self-esteem on their appearance. Losing one's hair is devastating for most people. Michelle focuses on helping women with hair loss feel better about themselves. She influences them to embrace their natural beauty, and help them to realize that they have different hair replacement options available to them. If anyone suffering from hair loss is looking for support, a listening ear, a shoulder to (virtually) cry on, she is here. Please reach out to her via social media @ladybehindthewig or visit her website at www.ladybehindthewig.com

Lorna Mastin While many may feel that they need more money, more time or more resources to make their dreams come true, she knows firsthand that without a mindset shift, those things won't matter. As a coach, mentor and doula to women of all ages, Lorna Mastin is best known for guiding women through changing their mind—ushering them from a place of poverty, to personal purpose and prosperity. Where others often see destitution and desperation, Lorna has mastered bringing out the best in others. Her strategic gift for uncovering and growing other people's gifts, talents and visions continues to open doors for her in both public and private sectors—further positioning her as an expert amongst the competition. Unlike other leaders, who are often taught or trained to lead over time, it was evident early on in life that she was a natural born leader. Her innate ability to solve problems, offer wisdom and insight beyond her years, and pull greatness out of others that they didn't see within themselves didn't just make her a success at Big Brothers, Big Sisters. It set her up for success in life in general. For Lorna, "Where there's a will, there's a way" isn't just a catchy slogan. It's a lifestyle. After overcoming low self-esteem and suicidal thoughts, she learned the true power of the mind and the mouth, igniting the passion within to redefine the mind of women worldwide. That passion unlocked unlimited opportunities for growth and expansion in both her personal and professional life. She is a mentor for the National Alopecia Areata Foundation. In addition to serving as program director for the Daughters of Citadel mentoring group, Lorna also served as YASC president and advisor for years. As a former strategic coordinator intern for NLC Consultants, she also planned and hosted events for celebrities and professional athletes. Holding both a certification in Massage Therapy and Life Coaching. She earned a Bachelor of Kinesiology, and obtained her Master's degree in Sports Administration. Through her nonprofit organization, Priceless Rubies, she encourages and empowers women to be the best version of themselves—in business, family, finances and relationships. Whether she's hosting a fitness fun event, comedy show fundraiser, her Annual Project Redefined, or giving back to the community, she has the drive and tenacity to simply get things done where others see impossibility. Offering workshops and programs that equip attendees with the necessary tools for success, her extensive arsenal of resources and connections makes winning easy for even the beginning entrepreneur or budding student. For more information or booking, visit www.pricelessrubies.com or email pricelessrubies88@gmail.com

Shay Bolling is a thirty-three-year old hairstylist & entrepreneur in Sacramento, California. She currently does hair and has a vision to launch her own hairline in January 2021, with the bigger vision of making wigs for women who suffer from hair loss, be if from cancer, alopecia, or any kind of hair loss. She would like to eventually be able to give back to her city and around the world to teenage girls who can't afford quality hair services. "My vision is indeed bigger than me!" Shay decided to be a hairstylist because she loved having the ability of connecting with women from many different walks of life and making them feel beautiful through the power of hair. Contact Shay by sending an email to southernbaby2009@gmail.com.

Uniqua Sade Leak was born May 6, 1991 in Detroit Michigan. She graduated from Consortium College Preparatory high school in 2009. Leak certified in 2010 as a Nursing Assistant from Henry Ford Community College. By 2013 Uniqua had become a registered Medical assistant through Kaplan Career Institute. She has been commissioned to numerous nursing facilities and hospitals throughout the Metro-Detroit with pride. In the summer of 2017, Uniqua earned her Associates of Arts from Wayne County Community College district and currently serves as a Medical Assistant Instructor and float ER Technician. The medical field is a difficult career, but Leak says "it's what I love to do". Uniqua keeps herself busy, she opened an organic body product line (UniquelyU). After having two children, Uniqua learned the importance of "knowing her rights as a women." She decided to start her own Birth and postpartum Doula company (Unique Doula Services) to serve teen moms and other women in need of a support partner. She currently attends Wayne State University and is majoring in Public health. Uniqua hopes to work in infectious disease in the near future. Uniqua is an Alopecia advocate, Warrior, and sister.

For more information: Uniqua.leak@gmail.com
Facebook: Uniqua Leak
Instagram: @Sadeuniquee2 and @uniquedoulaservices

Tamara Flake, is the visionary behind the brand iRockitBald. This organization began as a social media handle on Instagram in 2012. The brand took off in September of 2016 when Tamara began going live telling her alopecia story for Alopecia Awareness Month. Since then, iRockitBald has been featured in the Hats off Alopecia Fashion Shows, Bald Beautiful and Bold Fashion Show, The Keep Smiling Movement – Bald Beautiful and Bold Edition, Fear of Oxygen Documentary, Bald Life Magazine, The William Malcolm Show, multiple radio shows and speaking engagements throughout the city of Detroit.

The primary mission of iRockitBald is to uplift individuals living with hair loss due to alopecia at whatever point in their journey they may be. It is the mission of iRockitBald to encourage those living with alopecia to embrace their truth, build strength and courage through loving yourself. To support you through the transition and process of Rocking It Bald or not. The primary focus is building self-love and confidence.

The vision of iRockitBald is to educate, encourage, motivate and uplift individuals living with or loving someone with hair loss. We desire to connect individuals to medical professionals and resources i.e., dermatologist, endocrinologists, psychologists through online platforms and by hosting meet and greets, community awareness events, seminars, webinars, fundraisers, walks, parties, fashion shows, trips, conferences, and virtual events.

If you are someone struggling with an alopecia diagnosis or hair loss, we recommend you take some time to self-assess and identify what you love about you. Self-love is the number one key. Then surround yourself with people who care for you unconditionally and support your truth. Surround yourself with likeminded individuals; seek them out socially at in person events or via social media. Educate yourself, know your worth and do what makes you feel your best. Most importantly, it is your process. Take as long as you need to grow through it.

For more information or booking please visit www.irockitbald.com or email irockitbald@gmail.com.

Raquel Johnson is fifty years old born in Benton Harbor, Michigan, and raised in Detroit. She has one son who is thirty-three and one grandson who is twelve. She has been employed by Blue Cross Blue Shield of Michigan for twenty-two years, and she is currently a senior analyst. She has Bachelors in Business Leadership and Masters in Health Care Administration.

You may contact her at Rdennis88@yahoo.com. Her favorite scripture is Romans 8:38-39.

Charlene Stewart was born in Mobile, Alabama, in 1971. She married Ron Stewart in 1990. She is a mother of five children with three grandkids & one on the way. She has worked as a nurse for the past seventeen years, and is looking to exceed that for as long as God sees fit.

Curtis Motley lives in Jacksonville, Florida. He was born and raised in Akron, Ohio. He and his wife have been married for thirty-five years. His hobbies are bowling, fishing and a good game of dominoes.

He survived COVID-19 and shares his story in *Confinement Chronicles* in order to encourage others.

Tracy Etheridge, is a beautiful, bold, bald Runway Model who has an autoimmune disorder called Alopecia. She loves to travel, meet new people, and Rip, Slay, and Demolish the Runways all over the World. Tracy is a radio host for WDRB media in Charlotte, North Carolina, and a TV host for Divas Studio Plus for the weekly show "My AIR." Tracy is also the Owner/CEO of Divas Boutique, an online retail boutique and the model group Runway Slayer Models.

Tracy RunwayModelDiva Etheridge
Email address: MyAIRwTracyEtheridge@gmail.com
Website: Divasboutique.shop
FB: My AIR TV/Radio Show - Tracy RunwayModeldiva Etheridge
    Divas Boutique - Runway Model Diva
IG: Runwaymodeldiva - DivasBoitiqueshop MyAIRTracy

YouTube: My A.I.R. Tracy Etheridge

Chaconna Downs uses her love for Christ and gift of encouragement as the dynamic duo for ministry. Coming from a large but close-knit family only fueled her passion and created a desire to see broken people and families restored, healed, and made whole.

In 2012 she earned her Masters of Social Work from Asbury University. At the same time, Chaconna was under the leadership and training of Pastor Larry Weathers to become a licensed, ordained minister and pastor. Later that year, she, along with a team of ministers from The Revolution Mark 16:20, would go on to plant and co-pastor the Berea location of the ministry. A burden for taking Jesus outside the four walls was the seed that grew Loved Right Ministries. The ministry modeled in servant-leadership launched in 2014, with the sole purpose of meeting people right where they are to share the love of Christ.

Relocation to Daytona Beach birthed her first published book, *Simple Sayings: Sprinkles of Encouragement.* A new ministry assignment would be the catalyst for the next two books and #UntilHeArrives, the singles ministry that she now pastors. Chaconna is blessed to share her gifts in Central Florida and abroad through books, workshops, blogging, and public speaking.

Chad Butler shares that he is forty years old, an entrepreneur that owns several businesses, and works as an independent contractor for a delivery service. He is Michigan resident educated through the School of Life, a father, and a husband. He may be reached via email:
sonyabennett.author@gmail.com for privacy purposes.

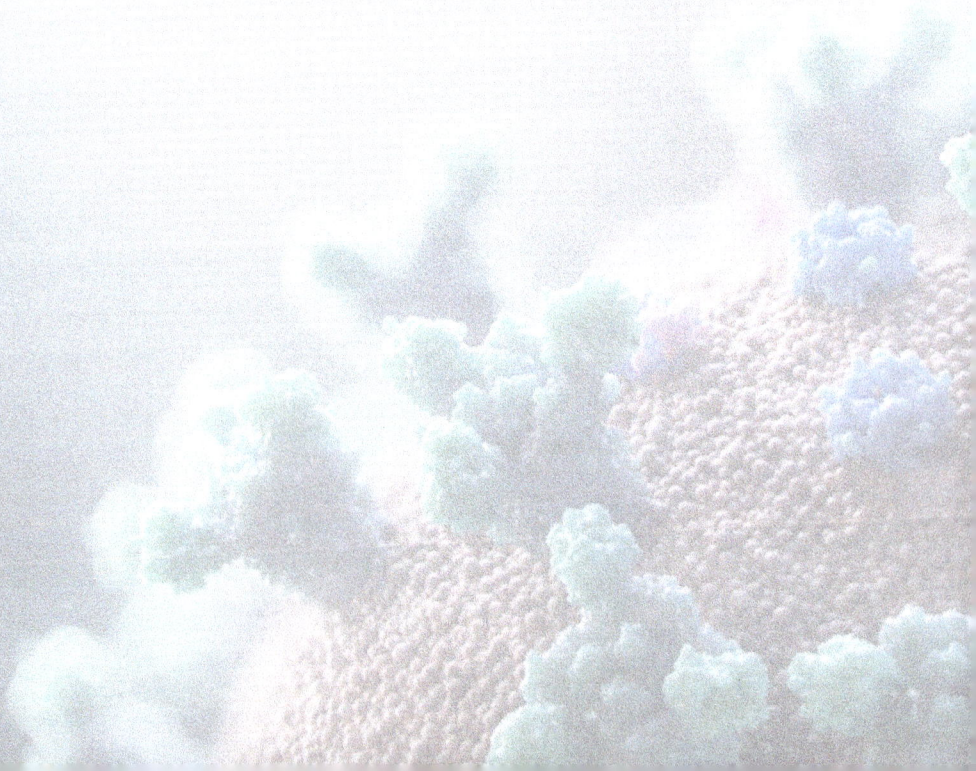

PROMOTIONAL SPONSOR

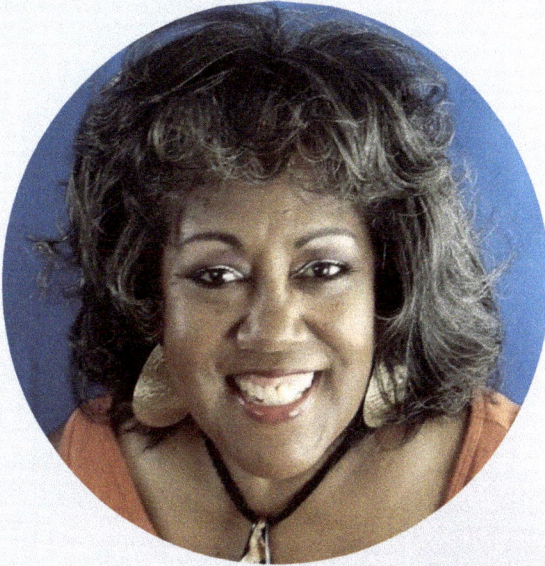

Special thanks to our promotional sponsor, The F.R.E.S.H. BOOK FESTIVAL™. The founder of the festival is Author Donna Gray-Banks, and she sends out an email blast, introducing her readers and followers to each volume in the *Confinement Chronicles* series.

Learn more online about one of the largest book festivals in Florida by visiting www.FRESHbookFestivals.net, and we hope to see you there, in January!

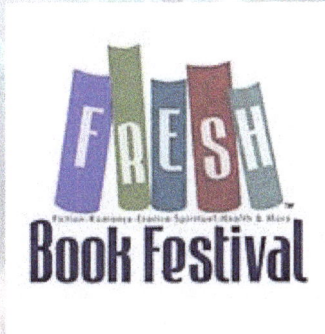

PROMOTIONAL SPONSOR

Triumphant Magazine

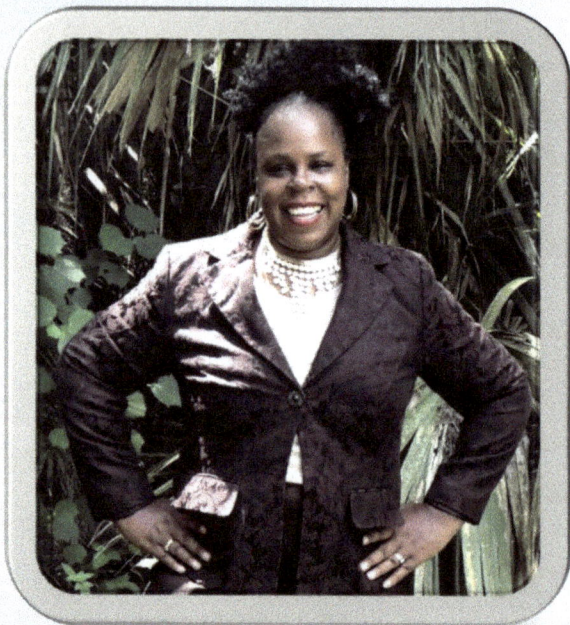

Theresa Jordan is the Founder of *Triumphant Magazine*, and she is the founder of Jordan Destinations Travel & Event Planning. Theresa resides in Florida, and she is a phenomenal entrepreneur. The good Lord pushed her out of the corporate world, September 2016, and He has blessed her gigantic opportunities since He closed those doors. He continues to show her that He is a promise keeper, and He remains to be faithful. Her motto is everything that has happened to her that was good, it was because "God Did It."

Theresa is a contributing author to *Confinement Chronicles* produced by Angie BEE Productions & *Daily Dose of Declarations* by Melanie Bonita Enterprises.

Theresa is a contributing Motivational Speaker, a speaker for Women's Conferences and the founder of Sisters Encouraging Sisters.

Follow us online www.Facebook.com/TriumphantMagazine and visit www.TriumphantMagazine.com

On behalf of all of the authors featured in *Confinement Chronicles*, and Angie BEE Productions, we would like to thank Theresa Jordan for featuring us in the pages of *Triumphant Magazine*.

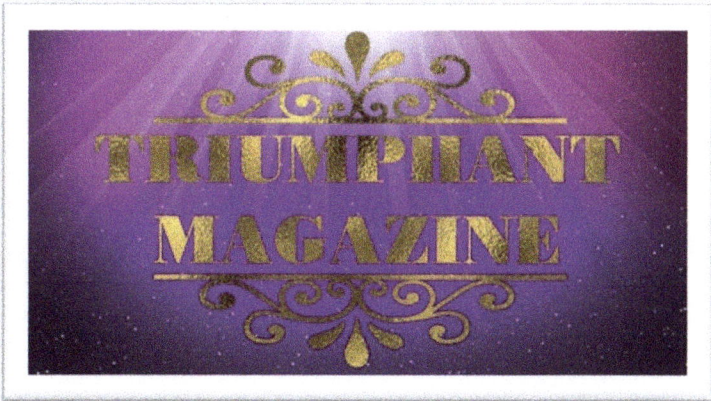

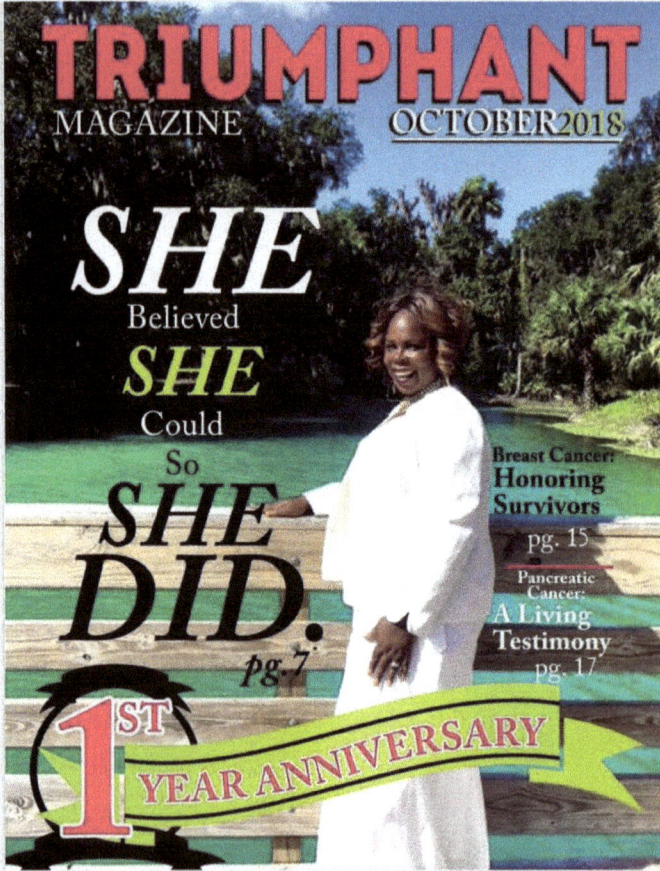

TRIUMPHANT
MAGAZINE   OCTOBER 2018

SHE
Believed
SHE
Could
So
SHE
DID.
pg. 7

Breast Cancer:
Honoring
Survivors
pg. 15

Pancreatic
Cancer:
A Living
Testimony
pg. 17

1ST
YEAR ANNIVERSARY

**DETAILS ABOUT THE MUSIC IN
THE AUDIOBOOK VERSION**

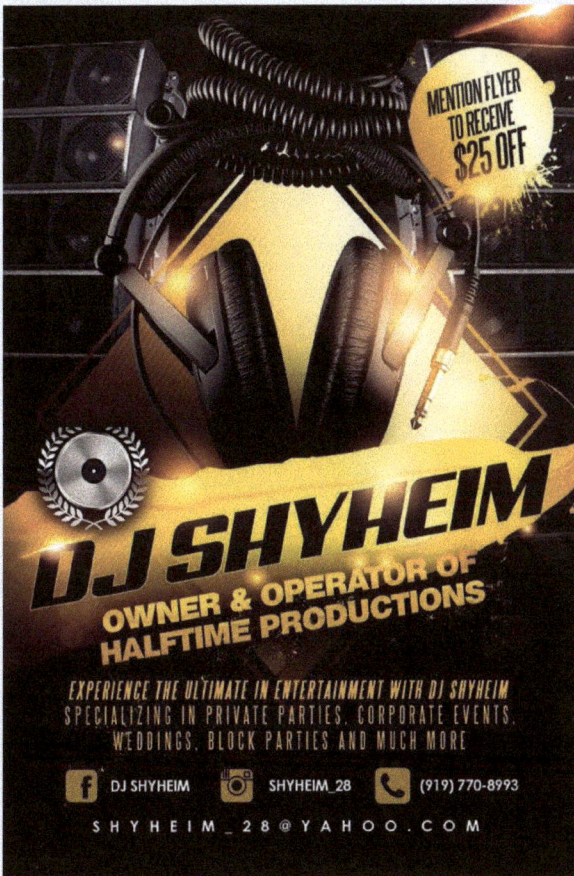

The background music that is heard in the audiobook version of *Confinement Chronicles* is produced by the incomparable Larry D. Boyd, also known as DJ Shyheim. I live in North Carolina, and this is where I am reputable for my professional Disc Jockey services. Check out my homepage for more detailed information about what I do. Keep reading the text provided on this page to get familiar with my story and how I became a DJ.

PROFESSIONAL AND RELIABLE
WEDDING & BIRTHDAY PARTY DISC JOCKEY SERVICES IN
NORTH CAROLINA

When I was in high school, I used to stay up late at night recording all the trending songs on the radio. I kept doing that until it became my profession. I have performed in Japan, Florida, and California, working with major artists such as Christian (on Roc-A-Fella Records), and as a DJ for Goodie Mob, Bad Azz, and others.

I personally believe that bringing a different sound to the table is the most important part of the job. Artists should be taken aside and compared to others. This is what I offer here at Halftime Productions – a unique sound and professional Disc Jockey service suitable for every event.

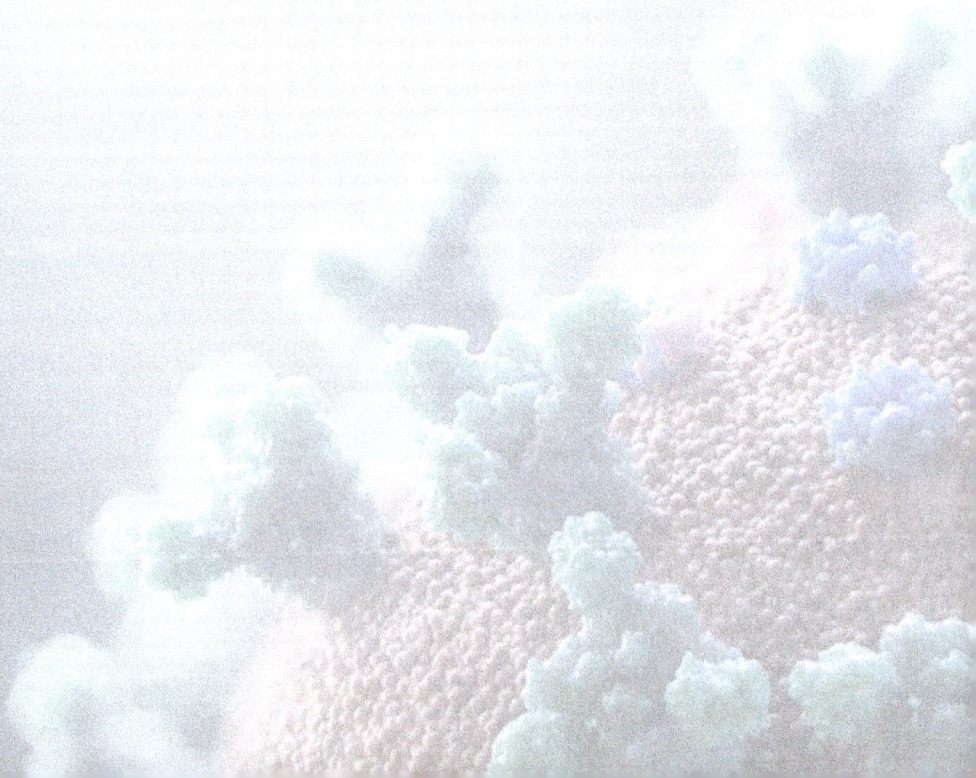

WHY CHOOSE ME?

**Nearly 20 years of Experience ~ Pure Dedication
Qualification ~ Professional Equipment ~ Reasonable Rates**

CALL (919) 770-8993 WHENEVER YOU NEED OUR
PROFESSIONAL DISC JOCKEY SERVICE IN NORTH
CAROLINA!

If you are planning a special event in or around the NC area and looking for an experienced DJ to contact, know that you are making the right choice with me. Call Halftime Productions now at (919) 770-8993 to check for availability!

Website: http://halftimeproductionsnc.com/
Email: shyheim_28@yahoo.com

Instagram
shyheim_28

Facebook
djshyheim

Twitter
djshyheim

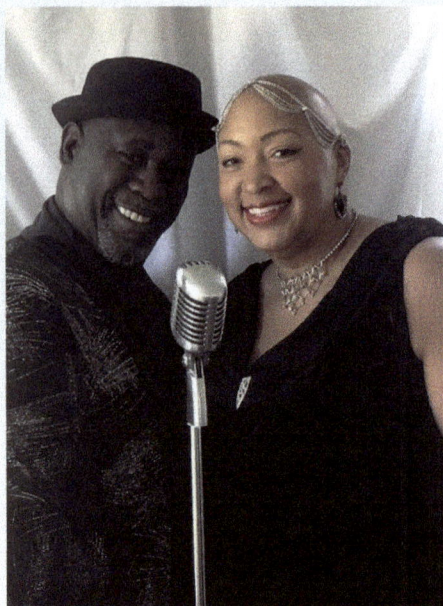

Evangelist Angie BEE preaches from a prophetic gift from God. She conducts red carpet event interviews and features those videos on her page at Facebook.com/AngieBEEpresents.

After retiring from a decade as an award-winning global radio show host, she now uses her anointed voice to narrate and produce audio books for authors and publishing companies.

Angie BEE is a Mental Health Advocate and motivational speaker and she is a recipient of several community awards for her participation and leadership.

Bartee is well sought after throughout Central Florida and is referred to as "The Rage of the Stage" because of his Smooth Jazz, Motown Review, and Vintage Soul musical performances.

He leads the "Dads-on-Duty" ministry workshop, brings "Movies Under The Stars with Bartee" to a variety of communities, and shares a powerful and loving testimony alongside Angie BEE during the "God, Me & You" marriage workshop and retreat.

Angie BEE & Bartee are authors. Whether they write solo works, together, or within collaborations, they are sure to have a book -- in print or audio -- that will bless you, help you, and inspire you.

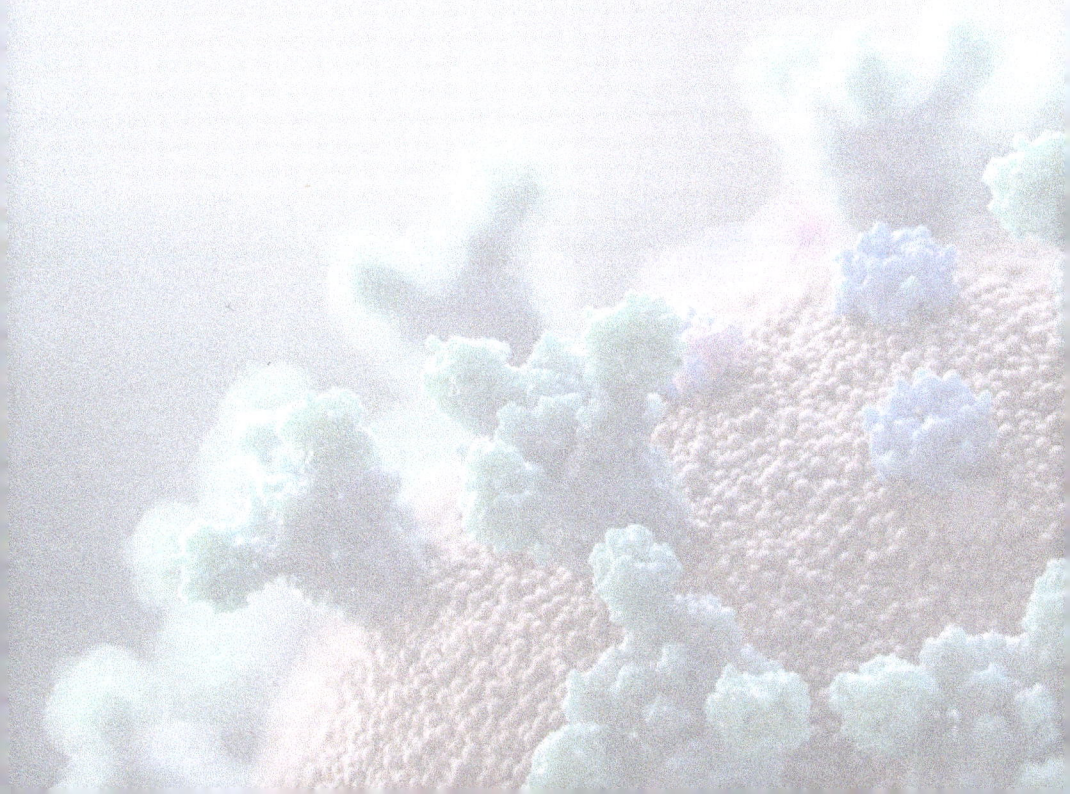

www.ingramcontent.com/pod-product-compliance
Lightning Source LLC
Chambersburg PA
CBHW052015030426
42335CB00026B/3161